The 3-Hour Diet™

How Low-Carb Diets Make You Fat and *Timing* Makes You Thin

Praise for Jorge Cruise's
The 3-Hour Diet™

"Feel like pasta for dinner? Not a problem. Some toast with those eggs? Bring it on. With Jorge's 3-Hour Diet™, eating great and losing weight has never been this simple."
—Jacqui Stafford, *Shape* magazine

●

"Combining cutting-edge research with practical how-to, Jorge Cruise's revolutionary approach to eating constitutes a sustainable way to slim down without sacrifice. Jorge offers up powerful kindling that can reignite the motivation of even the most jaded dieter. If you've always wanted a smart, caring weight-loss coach at your disposal 24/7, this book is for you!"
—Carol Brooks, editor in chief, *First for Women* magazine

●

"Jorge Cruise has identified a fundamental tenet of successful weight loss—that how you eat is just as important as what you eat. His 3-Hour Diet™ is easy to understand, simple to follow, and specifically designed for those who don't have time to diet. In short, his book is an essential tool for those seeking lifelong weight loss and maintenance."
—Lisa Sanders, MD, Yale University School of Medicine and author of *The Perfect Fit Diet*

●

"The 3-Hour Diet™ offers a simple nutrition prescription: how often and how much to control your hunger, *enjoy your food,* and *improve your health.* You can't get much better than that!"
—Leslie Bonci, MPH, RD, LDN, director of sports medicine nutrition, University of Pittsburgh Medical Center, and nutritionist for the Pittsburgh Steelers

●

"At last, the book to rival the Atkins and South Beach diets is here. If you want to lose weight and keep it off, without giving up any of the food groups, this is the book!"
—John Robbins, author of *Diet for a New America* and *The Food Revolution*

●

"Jorge has dedicated his life to showing people they can lose weight safely, and this book provides them with the skills to keep the weight off for life. It's a great plan and an inspiring book."
—Kathleen Daelemans, author of *Cooking Thin with Chef Kathleen* and *Getting Thin and Loving Food!*

●

"Jorge Cruise brings a new dimension to the world of weight loss—empowering and giving you the tools to lose weight by making simple changes in how and when you eat. This technique can help make all the difference."
—Fred Pescatore, MD, author of *The Hamptons Diet* and former associate medical director at the Atkins Center

●

"Jorge Cruise will keep you looking and feeling your best."
—David Kirsch, author of *The Ultimate New York Body Plan*

"Jorge's 3-Hour Diet™ offers a sound and practical eating plan. His easy-to-follow guide will help any follower see immediate body transformations with long-lasting results."
—Tammy Lakatos Shames and Lyssie Lakatos, RD, LD, CDN, authors of
Fire Up Your Metabolism

●

"Wow! I learned a lot from Jorge's fascinating new book. I can easily see how people who follow the 3-Hour Diet™ can shed pounds by keeping their fat-burning metabolism revved up."
—Lucy Beale, author of *The Complete Idiot's Guide to Weight Loss*

●

"An easy alternative to low-carb, high-fat, or other diets that can have harmful side effects."
—Dale Eustace, PhD, professor of cereal technology, Kansas State University

●

"This simple, easy-to-understand book gives you practical ideas that you can use immediately to lose weight without feeling hungry, without counting calories, and without feeling deprived in any way. I suggest you get one copy for yourself and one for a friend so you can enjoy the process together."
—Christopher Guerriero, founder and chairman of the National Metabolic and Longevity Research Center and author of *Maximize Your Metabolism*

●

"It's refreshing to hear a popular weight-loss guru pan low-carb and other fad diets and tell people the truth: that they can eat anything in moderation. The plan is nutritionally balanced, smart, and practical. The tone is encouraging and forgiving."
—Janis Jibrin, MS, RD, writer for GoodHousekeeping.com, and author of *The Unofficial Guide to Dieting Safely*

●

"The 3-Hour Diet™ will help millions lose weight and feel great! Eating healthy foods every three hours can help stabilize blood sugar levels, stave off hunger, and melt away unwanted pounds."
—Jay Robb, certified clinical nutritionist and author of *The Fat Burning Diet*

●

"Jorge does a great job of creating a straightforward, easy-to-follow eating plan that does not sound like a prison sentence! No restricting carbs, no exotic supplements, and no complex math calculations to make before every meal. *The 3-Hour Diet™* is easy to read and simple to follow!"
—Harley Pasternak M.Sc., celebrity trainer, and author of *Five Factor Fitness*

●

"The goal in life is to get more done in less time, and Jorge Cruise teaches you how to lose the weight you want in a healthy, safe way in *The 3-Hour Diet™*. What could be better? This is a book that can get you to your physical fitness goal in the shortest, easiest, best way ever."
—Mark Victor Hansen, cocreator, #1 *New York Times* best-selling series *Chicken Soup for the Soul®*, coauthor, *The One Minute Millionaire*

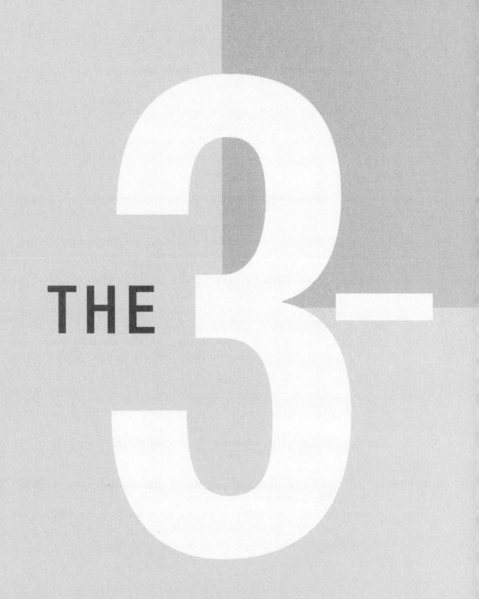

THE 3-

Hour Diet™

How Low-Carb Diets Make You Fat and *Timing* Makes You Thin

Jorge Cruise

New York Times Best-selling Author
and AOL Weight-Loss Coach

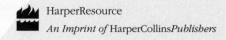
HarperResource
An Imprint of HarperCollins*Publishers*

The information given here is designed to help you make informed decisions about your body and health. The suggestions for specific foods, nutritional supplements, and exercises in this program are not intended to replace appropriate or necessary medical care. Before starting any exercise program, always see your physician. If you have specific medical symptoms, consult your physician immediately. If any recommendations given in this program contradict your physician's advice, be sure to consult your doctor before proceeding. Mention of specific products, companies, organizations, or authorities in this book does not imply endorsement by the author or the publisher, nor does mention of specific companies, organizations, or authorities in the book imply that they endorse the book. The author and the publisher disclaim any liability or loss, personal or otherwise, resulting from the procedures in this program. Internet addresses and telephone numbers given in this book were accurate at the time the book went to press.

Product pictures, trademarks, and trademark names are used throughout the book to describe and inform the reader about various proprietary products that are owned by others. No endorsement of the information contained in this book has been given by the owners of such products and trademarks, and no such endorsement is implied by the inclusion of product pictures or trademarks in this book.

Jorge Cruise, 3-Hour Diet, 3-Hour Plate, 3-Hour Timeline, 8 Minute Moves, 8 Minutes in the Morning, Visual Timing, and Weight Loss for Busy People are trademarks of JorgeCruise.com, Inc., and may not be used without permission.

HarperCollins books may be purchased for educational, business, or sales promotional use. For information please write: Special Markets Department, HarperCollins Publishers Inc., 10 East 53rd Street, New York, NY 10022.

FIRST EDITION

Designed by Ellen Cipriano

Jacket photograph copyright © by Scott Gries, Getty Images
Use of the Rubik's Cube® is by permission of Seven Towns Ltd
First for Women magazine cover on page 200 used with permission by Bauer Publishing Group

Library of Congress Cataloging-in-Publication Data

Cruise, Jorge.
    The 3-hour diet: how low-carb diets make you fat and *timing* makes you thin / by Jorge Cruise.—1st ed.
        p. cm.
    Includes bibliographical references and index.
    ISBN 0-06-079229-9
    1. Reducing diets. I. Title.

RM222.2.C768   2005
613.2'5—dc22   2004060686

05 06 07 08 09 WBC/RRD 10 9 8 7 6 5 4 3 2 1

To my three million online clients at JorgeCruise.com who requested that I create a realistic, simple, and healthy diet plan for *busy* people.

CONTENTS

ACKNOWLEDGMENTS

First, I want to thank my three-million-and-growing weight-loss clients at JorgeCruise.com whom I have had the privilege of coaching. Without their feedback, insight, and support, the 3-Hour Diet™ would not be the success it is today.

To Dr. David Katz, the true role model for all doctors. Your message of integrative medicine is extremely powerful. The world is extremely fortunate to have your message, and luckier that you are such a passionate and extraordinary messenger as well. I look forward to many projects together. Thanks, David, for being my inspiration as a true health pioneer as well as a great husband and father to your family. Bravo!

I must thank Oprah Winfrey, the lady who launched my career. She invited me to be a guest on her show in Chicago and introduced me to two people whose lives had changed because of my Web site. I will never forget that day. From that moment on, I knew that the Internet was a powerful resource that could change people's lives and bodies.

Heather, my wife, whom I love so much. Thanks for being my best friend and the center of my life. You have brought balance and fun into my life. My life truly started when we met. Thank you so much, baby doll. I am so grateful—you are my girl.

To my son, Parker. Thank you so much, buddy, for making me smile every day and for all the happiness you have brought into my life. I am a very lucky daddy.

Ben Gage, my company president and legal ace. Thanks for all your efforts and support. I look forward to a lifetime of empowering America with you.

To Phyllis McClanahan and Jenn Anderson. Thank you both for running the home office. And an extra big thank you for your extraordinary efforts and support on this book. I am the luckiest man to be surrounded by such smart women. Thank you for your loyalty and belief that we can change the world. I cannot imagine my life without you both. Thank you, thank you, thank you!

To my advisory circle. Thank you Halle Elbling, MS, RD, Vanessa Aldaz, MPH, RD, Linda Spangle, RN, MA, Janette J. Gray, MD, Cory Baker, CPT, NASM, Chef Bernard Guillas, Andrew Roorda, MD, and Jade Beutler, supplement expert. I am so grateful for your time, efforts, and friendship. Thanks so much!

To my sister, Marta, for her love. And of course to my beautiful Mama, Gloria, and her many sacrifices that allow me to stand where I am today. Plus a big thank you to my mom-in-law, Sue, for all her help with the refining of this book too. I am lucky to have a mom-in-law that is a true master of words and loves us so much (congrats on your weight loss too)!

To Cathy Leavy for her extraordinary design of the 3-Hour Plate™ and the 3-Hour Timeline™.

To Lisa Sharkey, my friend who has a heart of gold.

To Cristina Saralegui, the best adopted mom anyone can ever have. Besitos.

Thank you Scott Gries for your extraordinary talent with the cover photograph.

To Jacqui Stafford who is a diva of style and good taste. Thank you for your support with all that I do. You are a true gem.

To Bruce Barlean and the whole Barleans family. Thanks for everything.

To my buddy and great friend Jade Beutler and his family.

To all my friends at AOL, *First for Women* magazine, and *USA Weekend*.

To Steve Hanselman, the man at HarperCollins whose passion and vision for *The 3-Hour Diet™* made this revolution a reality. Thank you Steve for your friendship and extraordinary support.

And of course to my outstanding team at HarperCollins who breathes life every day into the 3-Hour Revolution. Thank you Jane Friedman, Brian Murray, Joe Tessitore, and George Bick. Thank you so much Kathryn Huck, Shelby Meizlik, Tara Cibelli, Shakti Shukla, Josh Marwell, René Alegría, Mary Ellen Curley, Laura Ingman, and Sabrina Ravipinto. Thank you all so much!

FOREWORD

by David L. Katz, MD
Yale University School of Medicine

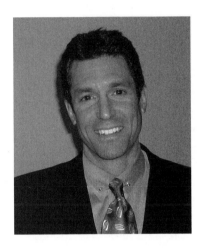

J orge Cruise understands weight control. He knows that losing weight
quickly is relatively easy, but that gaining it back with interest just as
quickly is both predictable and devastating. He knows a fad when he
sees one.

In fact, the one word I would choose to represent my friend and col-
league to you is *understanding*. Jorge will guide you to both weight loss
and lasting weight control with an incomparable wealth of understanding.
He has done his homework, so he understands human metabolism. He understands the science of nutrition, the fundamentals of physiology. But
what really sets Jorge apart is that he understands you! He communicates
regularly with several million clients at www.JorgeCruise.com. He gets insight and feedback from the more than twenty-three million he advises on
nutrition at America Online. He has been everywhere, talked to everyone,
and listened with genuine interest, concern, and rare empathy. Jorge understands weight loss.

The 3-Hour Diet™ is the product of that understanding. **This book will**

unquestionably help you lose weight and keep it off, because it is written by somebody who understands what it takes to get that job done. Jorge knows that cutting out whole categories of food from your diet can't last. Most of us rebel against such restrictions, and pay the price when we do. He knows as well that even if restrictive fad diets could be maintained, they would still be a bad idea, because they are at odds with health. Jorge will guide you to weight loss, but not at the price of your health.

In *The 3-Hour Diet*™, Jorge places a primary emphasis on the timing of food intake. This is a powerful insight. Eating in accord with this plan offers both physiological and psychological benefits. You will never need to be hungry, so there is no sense of deprivation. You do not need to jettison whole categories of food to get calories under control. By spreading food out in frequent meals and snacks, you lower insulin levels, reducing the tendency to make body fat. The plan is even designed to help maximize your body muscle without exercise.

If I may have two words to describe Jorge, then I would add *caring* to understanding. Jorge Cruise doesn't just understand how to help you lose weight. He cares about how you get there!

Because of this caring, Jorge will not resort to deception or exaggerated sales pitches to gain your interest or attention. If you want to lose a pound a day, look elsewhere. Jorge is courageous enough to say—quite correctly—that you should not be losing more than about two pounds a week if you want your weight loss to be both safe and permanent. Jorge is also honest and correct in acknowledging that calories count, and all arguments to the contrary are smoke and mirrors.

Jorge Cruise has built *The 3-Hour Diet*™ on a foundation of deep understanding and genuine caring. To that can be added one more vital ingredient: experience. As you may already know, Jorge lived through, and nearly died from, his own struggles with weight and health. Yet he turned this situation around so thoroughly that he is now a role model of health and fitness for us all. Jorge is not sending you off to parts unknown; he is inviting you to follow a trail he has dutifully blazed.

The unique understanding, caring, and experience of Jorge Cruise come together in *The 3-Hour Diet*™. This book is a gift you can and should give yourself if lasting weight control eludes you. And if you are one of those rare individuals who has your own weight fully under control—congratulations! Give this book as a gift to someone you love so they can get there, too!

The 3-Hour Diet™ is sensible and simple, practical and powerful, innovative yet intuitive. In the challenging quest for lifelong weight control, there are few who can guide us with the understanding, caring, and experience of

Jorge Cruise. In *The 3-Hour Diet*™, Jorge has paved the way to a healthier, happier, slimmer you. Follow it. In this excellent book, he is extending to you his sure and steady hand. Take it!

Dr. David Katz is one of the nation's foremost authorities on nutrition, weight control, and the prevention of chronic disease, Dr. Katz is a board-certified specialist in both Internal Medicine and Preventive Medicine. He cofounded and directs Yale's Prevention Research Center, where he has been personally responsible for managing some $15 million in research funds. In addition to nearly seventy scientific papers, Dr. Katz has authored eight books to date. Among these are a well-respected textbook on nutrition for health professionals (*Nutrition in Clinical Practice;* Lippincott Williams & Wilkins, 2001), and *The Way to Eat* (Sourcebooks, Inc., 2002), a guide to the skills and strategies needed for weight control and better nutritional health for the whole family. Dr. Katz also offers a comprehensive personalized online diet at www.thewaytoeat.net. Nutrition columnist to *O, the Oprah* magazine, and a health consultant to ABC's *Good Morning America,* Dr. Katz is a frequent source of expert opinion for the news media. He and his wife, Catherine, live in Connecticut with their five children: Rebecca, 16; Corinda, 15; Valerie, 10; Natalia, 9; and Gabriel, 5.

FROM THE DESK OF JORGE CRUISE

Dear Friend,

I want to welcome you to *The 3-Hour Diet*™! If you are like me, you are a busy person and really don't have time to waste. You don't have time for complicated plans that are unrealistic and, worst of all, in the long term cause you to regain all the weight back . . . and more. This plan is based on my own journey with weight and the success of my three million online clients.

First of all there will be NO deprivation—meaning you can eat carbs; NO calorie counting, NO pills, NO surgeries, and NO required exercising. Bottom line, with my 3-Hour Diet™ there are no restrictions on food options, ever. I believe that is critical to successful weight loss because you will never need to cheat and thus sabotage your success. Because really, how long can you go without eating bread? But the real secret to the 3-Hour Diet™ is *when* you eat. You see, timing is the revolutionary concept that has been kept secret for years. Yes, timing is what will make your body thin!

For now, get ready to start losing two pounds each week by bringing back the joy of eating. It's time to lose!

Best wishes,

JORGECRUISE™

Jorge Cruise
Creator of *JorgeCruise.com*

PART 1

Time to Lose

ONE

THE KEY TO A SLIM BODY

efore I started Jorge's program, my weight was out of control. I looked in the mirror and saw a huge, short, fat person. I hated buying clothes. I was tired and had no energy. I started Jorge's plan and I have lost 56 pounds so far and dropped four sizes. This program has shown me that even with five kids and a busy schedule, I can succeed with weight loss. Best of all, I did not have to give up the foods that I like. This plan is simple to follow. Thanks, Jorge!"

—BRENDA JOHNSON—LOST 56 POUNDS

Today, 65 percent of all Americans are overweight. This isn't just an American problem. Half of the people who live in the UK are overweight, too. It's an epidemic. Despite the abundance of diet books, pills, and programs, people are getting fatter. Obviously, the current dieting regimens are not working. Consider these statistics:

- According to the Centers of Disease Control, more than 300,000 Americans die each year from obesity-related illness. This means

An Epidemic Out of Control

More than 300,000 Americans die each year from obesity-related illnesses—second only to the 400,000 who die from using tobacco products. Each day more than 800 Americans die from problems related to obesity.

Obesity Trends* Among U.S. Adults
BRFSS, 1985
(*BMI =30, or ~30 lbs overweight for 5' 4" woman)

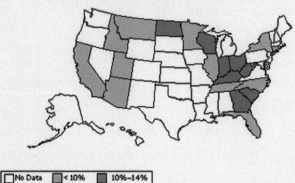

[ ] No Data   [ ] < 10%   [ ] 10%–14%

Obesity Trends* Among U.S. Adults
BRFSS, 2001
(*BMI =30, or ~30 lbs overweight for 5' 4" woman)

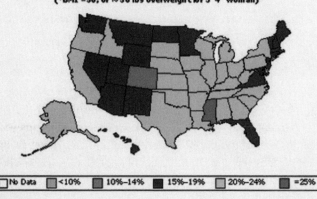

[ ] No Data   [ ] <10%   [ ] 10%–14%   [ ] 15%–19%   [ ] 20%–24%   [ ] =25%

SOURCE: CDC

each day more than 800 Americans die from problems related to obesity. This means every 5 minutes 3 people die.

- Twenty years ago, only 4 percent of American children were overweight. Today, that number has swelled to 15 percent—and it's growing larger by the day.
- On average, research shows Americans are *gaining* 1 to 2 pounds a year. Nine out of ten people who lose weight on a fad diet gain it all back within a year.

So here's the question: "Why are you unable to successfully lose and keep the weight off?" I wanted to know the answer to this question. So I studied the effects of many different diets and questioned thousands of my most successful online clients.

This is what I learned. Do you want to know why YOU can't lose weight and keep it off? Well, you won't find the answer in a low-carbohydrate diet, a grapefruit diet, a cabbage soup diet, or any other fad diet. Yep, it's not there. In fact, these diets actually make you fatter in the *long term*. (You'll learn more about why and how in chapters 2 and 3.) Starving yourself and cutting out your favorite foods never works. If you've ever tried such deprivation diets, you know this already. With every fad diet you tried, you may have lost weight, only to hit a plateau and then gain it all back and more too.

Indeed, the answer lies in something much simpler, much easier to implement in your life, and much more enjoyable to tackle. It lies in a dieting secret that has worked for many years for my most successful online clients—and for many other people as well. When I studied my most successful clients, I learned that the secret to dieting success lies in a revolutionary concept: *timing*. Yes, timing. You see, the secret to losing weight and keeping it off has to do with much more than what you eat. It centers on *when* you eat.

Specifically, it's not allowing more than 3 hours to pass without eating. Not every 5 hours or every 2 hours, but rather ideally every 3 hours. **Why every 3 hours?** Research study after research study confirmed the power of 3 hours. You see, if you allow more than 3 hours to pass between meals, your body turns on its natural "starvation protection mechanism," what I call your SPM. When your body's SPM gets switched on, your body thinks that it's in a famine. When this happens, your body does everything it can to preserve the most calorie-rich tissue in the body to ensure your survival. That tissue is body *fat*. Yes, your body begins to store fat and consumes precious fat-burning muscle instead. So now you might be losing weight on the scale, but you're not losing the ideal kind of weight. You're losing muscle instead of fat.

Height: 5'5"
Age: 52
Starting weight: 264 lbs.
Current weight: 157 lbs.
Other: Widowed full-time kindergarten
teacher with two adult children

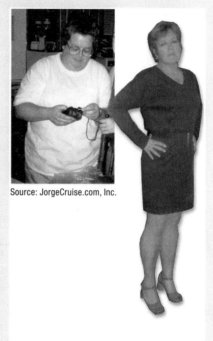

Source: JorgeCruise.com, Inc.

"Before the 3-Hour Diet™, I was a very fluffy, unfit woman. I had sad eyes and rarely smiled. I looked ten to fifteen years older than I really was. I wore baggy, unflattering clothes, didn't take much pride in my appearance, and wore no makeup. Of course, I wished I could change, but that was all I did—wish.

"Now that I've lost 107 pounds on the 3-Hour Diet™, I am a very self-confident woman, a woman who is in control. My eyes sparkle and I smile all the time. I look ten to fifteen years younger than I am. I am lean and toned. I look healthy. I wear clothing that shows off my hard work, and I feel as comfortable in a miniskirt or low-rise jeans as I used to in my loose sweats. I now wear a flattering hairstyle and makeup. When I look in the mirror, I see a size-8, 157-pound woman who looks vaguely familiar. Hey, that woman is me!"

Debbie's Secrets to Success:

- ➤ Make yourself your #1 priority.
- ➤ Plan your menus for a week at a time.
- ➤ Be prepared! Pack lunches the night before; cook chicken breasts ahead for the week; clean and cut up veggies before storing them.
- ➤ Keep one outfit in your previous clothing size visible—and swear to never wear it again.
- ➤ Keep a journal so you can see just how far you have come!
- ➤ Accept compliments graciously. You deserve them!

Why is losing lean muscle bad? It burns fat. Lean muscle controls your resting metabolism. Yep, lean muscle controls how many calories you burn when doing nothing . . . when resting on the couch, driving your car, sitting at the computer, even when sleeping in your bed. Each pound of muscle burns approximately 50 calories every day just doing nothing. Lose just 5 pounds of muscle and your metabolism burns 250 calories less a day; in the course of just one year that will equal 26 pounds of new fat!

You see, the fat on your body is not the source of your problem. You may not like having the excess fat, but the fat is not to blame. It's only the symptom. The true problem is the loss of lean muscle tissue from years of poor meal timing (see chapter 5) and/or fad dieting (see chapters 2 and 3). And muscle loss equals a lowered resting metabolism and thus a life of chronic weight gain.

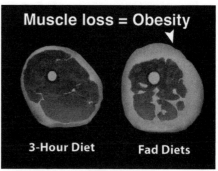

Muscle loss happens on most fad diets, as shown in these cross-sections of thighs (by magnetic resonance imaging). Source: JorgeCruise.com, Inc.

On the flip side, if you eat at the correct times, you "turn off" your body's SPM, which in turn encourages your body to burn fat without losing muscle. This preserves your resting metabolism and wham-o . . . you get and stay slim more easily!

You may be wondering, **"Is it just about eating every 3 hours? Is that all there is to this diet plan?" The answer is no. There is more. It's all about what I call _Visual Timing_™. What do I mean? Visual Timing™ has two secrets. It's all about creating an _automatic_ eating schedule by being visually aware of: 1) when to eat and 2) how to eat without restricting food options—ever.** Yep, you need to know how to easily eat without any restrictions on the food options you love. And my Visual Timing™ formula will ensure you eat automatically every 3 hours and not forget to eat. It will feel effortless. Depriving yourself of the foods you love leads to bingeing and failure in the long term. Chapters 5 and 6 will cover these two critical secrets. So get ready to stop thinking low-carb. Get ready to stop fad dieting. Get ready to start thinking about timing—_when_ you eat.

This new way of thinking will make weight loss effortless and, most important, sustainable. You'll finally be able to enjoy _what_ and _how_ you eat, and still lose weight. Bottom line, you will lose what doctors recommend as safe—2 pounds a week—by eating the foods you love. The best part of all: the weight will not come back.

Why Is 3 Hours the *Magic* Number?

Not only will eating every 3 hours turn off your "starvation protection mechanism" thus preserving precious fat-burning muscle and your resting metabolism, but there are more slimming reasons to eat every 3 hours:

- Increases your basal metabolic rate
- Increases your energy levels
- Suppresses appetite naturally
- Lowers cholesterol levels
- Reduces the belly-bulging hormone cortisol

NOTE: For more detailed information on the extraordinary power of eating every 3 hours jump to chapter 5.

Does this sound exciting? Keep reading to join the 3-Hour Diet™ revolution.

Why I Created the 3-Hour Diet™

You might be thinking to yourself, "Jorge has probably never been fat. He has always been trim and lean. Right?" The answer is no. You see, I used to be an overweight kid and young man. I know what it's like firsthand to feel embarrassed by extra weight. I've been there. My dad has been there. My sister has been there, too. At one time, we were all fat and unhealthy.

I grew up in Southern California with a mom from Mexico City and a dad from Pennsylvania. Both sides of the family loved huge portions. I probably ate enough food for three kids. I got so chubby that my mom used to call me *el rey*, which in Spanish means "the king," and before long I looked more like King Arthur's table: round. By the time I was fifteen, I was a physical disaster.

The kids at school used to call me "lard ass" or "fatso." Yeah, kids were mean to say the least. Junior high probably marked my worst years. I remember feeling humiliated during gym class when the captains would pick which kids would end up on their teams. I would hear them say, "I pick you," "you," "you," as student after student around me got picked for a team. As one student after another went to one of the teams, fewer and fewer stood around me, until no one else was left. I could see and hear the students snickering. No one wanted me to be on their team.

Because of my weight and asthma, I could never keep up. When we had to run the mile in gym class, the other students passed me as I wheezed. I felt so fat and slow. Most of all, I felt embarrassed. I couldn't do one pull-up or one push-up. I couldn't even do a push-up with my knees on the floor. I know what it's like to feel humiliated by my body.

I had low energy and daily headaches. No one—certainly not my family— ever suspected that my health challenges were caused by the way I ate.

It was during this time, I went through a life-changing experience. My appendix burst and I almost died. During my slow and painful recovery, I started thinking a lot about being a healthier person. I wasn't sure how to get started, but I knew I wanted to change my current patterns and begin a new way of life.

When I was 18, not long after my appendix burst, something happened that made me realize how I could begin that new way of life. My dad was diagnosed with prostate cancer, and the doctors told him he had a year to live. My dad and I enrolled in an alternative health center program in San Diego as a last resort. I was mainly there as emotional support for dad, but what I learned changed my life. At the center, Dad and I learned all about nutrition. After we changed our diets, our health improved. Dad's cancer went into remission and my headaches disappeared. We both lost weight and felt more energetic.

Still, I struggled for years to maintain this new, healthy lifestyle. Sometimes willpower was not enough to keep me on track. Then, when I was in college, I attended a one-day seminar by Anthony Robbins (who is now a good friend and wrote the foreword to my very first book). During the event, Tony asked the audience, *"If you could do anything and not fail, what would it be?"* After thinking about it for a while, I thought, "I want 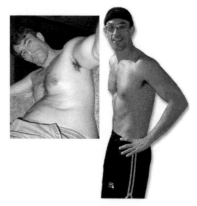 to get and stay healthy—and teach others how to do the same." **I realized that my health was most important—priority #1.** Without my health, nothing else was possible. I also realized that teaching others this important lesson would become my life's calling. That powerful lesson sent me on my life's journey: to be a weight-loss specialist for busy people.

The Real Consequence of Obesity

Overweight and obesity have been linked to numerous health problems, including diabetes, heart disease, and some types of cancer. A report in the *Journal of Science* predicts that obesity can shave as many as seven years off your life expectancy. Overweight and obesity have been linked to the following conditions:

- Premature death
- Hypertension
- Diabetes and insulin resistance
- Gall bladder disease
- Kidney disease
- Liver disease
- Heart disease
- Many types of cancer
- Arthritis
- Orthopedic disorders
- Fatal respiratory disease
- Stroke

- Gout
- Asthma
- Back pain
- Reproductive disorders in women
  menstrual disorders
  infertility
  miscarriage
  impaired fetal well-being
  diabetes mellitus during pregnancy
- Sleep apnea and snoring
- Chronic pain
- Depression

Since then I've been studying how to help people get healthy and lose weight. I've studied nutrition, exercise science, and communications at the University of California, San Diego (UCSD), Dartmouth College, and the Cooper Institute for Aerobics Research. I've also taken courses offered through the American College of Sports Medicine and the American Council on Exercise. I've purchased and read nearly every weight-loss book that has ever been published. And a few years ago, Arnold Schwarzenegger himself selected me to be part of his Physical Fitness Council in California, where I met one of my mentors in the diet and fitness world: Jack La Lanne. Since then I have also become good friends with some of the leading dieticians and physicians in the United States, including integrative medicine pioneers Dr. Andrew Weil of the University of Arizona and Dr. David Katz of Yale University. I've even formed an advisory circle of experts, whom I meet with regularly to discuss the latest health finds and trends (see pages 13–14).

I still have a scar to remind me of how lucky I am to be alive—and my determination to stay healthy. Today, I am a busy man. And I am also a husband and dad. And I have kept the weight off. Yep, I eat every 3 hours. And my wife Heather, who gave birth to our son, Parker, lost her pregnancy weight by eating every 3 hours, too. My zeal for weight control has inspired the rest of my family to get healthy too. They also stay slim by paying careful attention to when they eat.

My past is what started me on my life's work, but I created this book— The 3-Hour Diet™—in response to massive amounts of e-mail from people who visit my online diet center, JorgeCruise.com.

You see, in the past people usually came to visit me online after reading one of my *8 Minutes in the Morning*® books. These books are fitness plans based on restoring lean muscle via resistance training. They are excellent plans, but they require you to exercise. Consider them my "accelerated" plans for toning and firming, plans for when you don't just want to lose weight, but also want to get super-fit results.

And yet, countless numbers of the e-mails I got shared a common theme. People also wanted a healthy diet that worked, but that required little to *no exercise*. Such people told me they had no time to exercise. Some had many pounds to lose, and the excess weight made exercise too uncomfortable. Others had arthritis and other conditions that made their joints too painful to move comfortably. (Yes, imagine literally having over three million people e-mailing you.) They motivated me to take a step back. They all told me that sometimes they could not commit to exercising to lose weight, but of course they had to eat.

My heart told me that I had to create not a fitness-but diet-based plan that would be the first big step to help eliminate obesity. That's why I created the 3-Hour Diet,™ a simple diet that allows you to lose the weight and keep the weight off through good eating and with *no required exercising*.

How I Created This Book

I started my research by examining the most popular diets people use to lose weight. (Chapters 2 and 3 detail my findings about these diets.) I surveyed people visiting my site for the first time about the diets they'd tried in the past, asking them what worked and what did not. I did the same when I spoke at seminars or through my *First for Women* magazine column or through AOL as their exclusive weight-loss coach, and even when I traveled to London for book tours. I asked folks, "Have you been on a diet? Did you keep it off?" The answers were always the same: Yes, they had dieted, and No, the weight came back . . . plus more.

For every single diet, the story was the same. It did not deliver *lasting* results. Why? The diets were unrealistic and required too much willpower to follow. The dieters almost always ended up bingeing on ice cream or bread or whatever other food they had been restricting. And almost every single diet also eroded lean muscle, which directly destroyed the body's resting metabolism. And this was why so many times even before they fell off the dieting wagon—before they cheated—many dieters hit a plateau and then saw fat creep back onto their bellies, thighs, and hips. In many cases, most people regained more weight than they had lost! Remember that your muscle tissue is the single most important force behind a strong metabolism. Each pound of muscle burns 50 calories every day. Lose muscle and your metabolism starts to disappear.

So after discovering why various diets don't work, I set out to design a diet that *would* work. I wanted to create a diet that would not only help people to lose weight, but would also prevent muscle loss. I wanted to design a lasting plan, a diet that was easy to stick to, that people could maintain not only for one week or two weeks, but for the rest of their lives. My goal was to create a healthy way of eating that would make your body thin.

I knew from working with my online clients—and from the available scientific research—that cutting out entire food groups was not the answer. My advisory circle of experts and I had talked about it many times. Restricting carbs was not healthy. Restricting fat was not healthy. Restricting protein was not healthy. The human body needs carbohydrates, fats, and proteins. You should not restrict those food options—ever. I knew that a *healthy, sustainable* diet must include a balanced mix of carbohydrates, fats, and proteins in the right portions. I also knew that it must include treats and other foods that everyone loves, foods like chocolate. Including those foods was the only way to make the diet a lifelong journey rather than a short-term failure.

So I asked myself a question: "What was missing?"

That got me to focus on the research I had seen throughout the past few years. And what I saw was consistent: *timing* was essential. I discovered that the times people ate their meals was critical because it impacted the "starvation protection mechanism," which determined whether or not they could maintain their lean muscle mass and thus their metabolism.

So with that critical distinction, the feedback from my online clients and feedback from my advisory circle, I created the 3-Hour Diet.™ I tested the

HALLE ELBLING, MS, RD

Halle Elbling is an Associate Member of the American Dietic Association and Registered Dietician with a Masters in Nutritional Science from San Jose State University.

VANESSA J. ALDAZ, MPH, RD

Vanessa Aldaz is a Registered Dietician with a Masters in Public Health from Loma Linda University and Bachelor of Science in biochemistry and cell biology from the University of California San Diego.

JADE BEUTLER, SUPPLEMENT EXPERT

Jade Beutler is a nutritional supplement expert and the best-selling author of *Understanding Fats & Oils* and *Flax for Life!* He has devoted the last twenty years researching and developing lifestyle strategies to attain optimal health through sound dietary supplementation.

BERNARD GUILLAS, CHEF

Bernard Guillas began his culinary career when he arrived in the United States to work with former White House Chef Pierre Chambrin at the renowned Maison Blanche restaurant in Washington, DC. Today Chef Bernard is the head chef at the Marine Room in La Jolla, CA.

LINDA SPANGLE, RN, MA

Linda Spangle is the author of the nationally acclaimed book on emotional eating, *Life Is Hard, Food Is Easy.* Having personally struggled with food, Linda is passionate about helping individuals develop a level of peacefulness with food.

JANETTE J. GRAY, MD

Dr. Gray is a licensed internist and practices integrative medicine emphasizing prevention and embracing both conventional and holistic treatment options. She is the cofounder and medical director of The Center for Health and Wellbeing and attended medical school at the University of California, San Francisco.

ANDREW K. ROORDA, MD
Dr. Roorda currently resides in San Francisco and attended medical school at St. George's University School of Medicine. He completed his graduate work at Duquesne University and his undergraduate work at the University of California, San Diego.

CORY BAKER, CPT, NASM
Cory Baker is an exercise specialist certified by the National Academy of Sports Medicine and Apex Fitness Group. This knowledge, combined with her degree in communications from UCLA, gives a unique ability to share her fitness expertise easily with clients at all levels.

To contact any adviser, visit JorgeCruise.com.

plan with my online clients. I shared it with my advisory circle. And the results were phenomenal.

What You Can Expect

You will lose up to **two pounds a week** on the 3-Hour Diet™. You may be wondering why I promise just a 2-pound-a-week weight loss, whereas other popular diets claim you can lose 8 or more pounds in a week. Slow, steady weight loss allows your skin to slowly shrink along with your fat stores. This prevents the sagging skin that you sometimes see in people who have lost dramatic amounts of weight quickly. Slow, steady weight loss also gives you more energy. You'll be more likely to remain active, rather than feel worn out from your diet. Finally, you will never feel deprived or hungry, so you'll be less likely to binge and cheat. Plus you will **start losing belly fat first.** This is very important to my clients and I hope to you too. You see, you lower the stress hormone cortisol that is associated with stubborn belly fat (read more on page 58).

So there you have it: a diet plan that works long term, includes your favorite foods, and doesn't require exercise. My challenge to you right now is to commit to this program for four weeks. Take the plunge. You'll lose up to 2 pounds a week, lose belly fat first, and love the way you look.

It is time for you to lose!

TWO

WHY LOW-CARB DIETS MAKE YOU FAT

have not seen my face in over twenty years. I don't even know what I look like anymore. For years, all I saw was double chins and jowls. I also hated the rolls of fat around my middle. I had two kids and I lost the muscle tone in my abdomen. Well, guess what? My stomach has shrunk! And when I look in the mirror I am beginning to see a beautiful face looking back. Jorge's 3-Hour Diet™ is different from anything I've ever tried, and it works."

—TERESA NEAL LOST 25½ POUNDS

Short-term low-carb diets do produce weight loss. But, long term you will end up gaining the weight back and almost always will add new pounds, too. Bottom line is that low-carb diets will end up making you fat.

I know that may be hard for you to believe right now. You or many of your friends may be on low-carb diets—and some of them may even swear by them. Go to the supermarket and see aisle after aisle with one low-carb product after another. From bread to ice cream to soda—just about every product you can think of has now been modified for the low-carb lifestyle. That's not all. You may even have heard of some research—much talked about in the media—that low-carb diets don't harm your health, either.

All this may tempt you to run out and buy the latest low-carb diet book, throw all of your bread and pasta in the trash, and jump on the low-carb diet wagon. Well, don't be so fast to believe everything you see and hear about these diets. There's more to them than meets the eye (or mouth!).

How can I say low-carb diets will end up making you fat? How can I say low-carb diets are bad for your health? The answers to those questions lie in various university studies and in my own experience working with millions of online clients who, before they came to me, had tried just about every diet available—including low-carb diets.

Let me start by sharing with you a national network television investigative report I was involved in with *Dateline NBC*. The show picked six people who wanted to lose at least 30 pounds for their upcoming twenty-fifth high school reunion. The producers paired each person with a different weight-loss plan, pitting various diet plans against each other. They asked to have my plan as one of them. There I was competing against the Atkins® diet, hypnosis, Slim•Fast®, marathoning, and Weight Watchers®—all to see which method could result in the greatest weight loss within nine months.

I worked with the high school's former math club president, Eleanor Talbot. Over the next nine months I helped her to change the way she ate—conforming to the principles of the 3-Hour Diet™ and adding in my 8 Minute Moves® for firming and toning (you'll learn more about these optional metabolism-revving moves in chapter 11). Eleanor did very well, losing a stunning amount of weight. By reunion time, Eleanor was very happy with her results. By the end of our 9 months together, she had shed 60 pounds.

Although her weight loss was dramatic, she didn't lose as much as Rick Burnes, a U.S. Postal worker who lost 108 pounds on the Atkins® diet. Although the show initially showed him as the participant who lost the largest amount of weight, I wasn't concerned at the results. I knew the true winner would be revealed *after* the reunion, for I knew you may be able to lose weight faster on a low-carb diet, but it won't necessarily stay off for long—as the participants in the challenge soon learned.

The investigative program followed up with the weight-loss participants three months after the reunion. Eleanor was the only one who kept the weight off long term! Yep, everyone else in the weight-loss challenge had gained weight. Only Eleanor had kept it off. Interestingly, Burnes, the man on the Atkins® diet, regained the weight the fastest. He went off the diet the day after the reunion—putting back more than 50 pounds.

What about Eleanor? Not only was she the only one to not gain the weight back, but she was also the only one to lose *more*. She lost an additional 8 pounds in the three months following the reunion. She has now lost the most, 78 pounds, including those on Weight Watchers® or Slim•Fast®!

Why was Eleanor so successful? Eleanor followed my

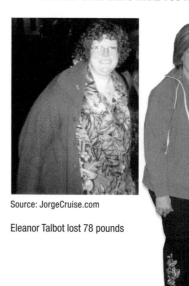

Source: JorgeCruise.com

Eleanor Talbot lost 78 pounds

eating recommendations of eating balanced meals every 3 hours. Rather than forgo entire food groups, Eleanor ate from all the food categories. At every meal, she included some carbohydrates, some protein, and even some fat. Each day she ate three meals, two snacks, and even one delicious treat. She included her favorite foods. She ate pasta, chocolate, and bread. Nothing was off-limits.

When I tell people this story, many of them ask me, "How could Eleanor lose so much weight and keep it off when she was not restricting carbs? How did she lose so much weight by eating chocolate—and bread?!"

The answer lies with what happened to her lean muscle tissue and thus her metabolism. You see, she did not lose lean muscle tissue. And you will recall that lean muscle determines how many calories you use at rest—your resting metabolism.

Eleanor preserved her lean muscle and thus preserved her resting metabolism by eating meals that included carbs every 3 hours. The Atkins® participant, on the other hand, had removed almost all carbs from his diet. And here is what happened to him whether he knew it or not: He lost lean muscle tissue and thus eroded his resting metabolism. Worse, he ended up craving the very foods he had eliminated from his diet. Once he reintroduced these foods, he overate them—consuming larger portions than his body could burn—and gained even more weight.

The bottom line is this: Anytime you go on a low-carb diet, you start to lose fat-burning lean muscle. Specifically, you erode muscle in three major ways:

A) Low-carb diets deplete sugar (glycogen) which is stored in your muscles.

B) Low-carb diets flush water out of your muscles.

C) Low-carb diets can cause fatigue and/or depression, which leads to a sedentary lifestyle. When you don't move, you lose muscle faster.

That's not all. In addition to lowering your metabolism, low-carb diets can spur weight gain in other ways. One is what I call "marketing misunderstanding." You see, too many people think that foods marketed as low-carb contain no calories. They think they can eat as much of them as they want and still lose weight. This simply isn't true. Calories are calories. Eat more than your body can burn and the excess gets stored in your fat cells. It's that simple. Worse, many of these low-carb products contain the same amount of calories as—if not more than—their higher-carb counterparts.

Finally, when you deprive yourself of carbs you will eventually binge on them. Yep, I have worked with three million online clients and I know that is a fact. Deprivation leads to bingeing and long-term failure.

Once you confidently walk away from low-carb diets, you will be able to finally stop losing lean muscle and thus stop the damage to your metabolism. Remember, every time you lose muscle your resting metabolism drops. Not only will you lose muscle in a low-carb diet, but there are other dangerous health risks such as constipation, bad breath, kidney and liver problems, heart disease and, for women, problems with conception. I hope once you read this chapter, you will also be able to share it with loved ones who are on a low-carb diet and help them make better choices, too. Now, let's get started with the full details.

Point 1: How low-carb diets derail your resting metabolism

There are a number of low-carb diets out there, all of them slightly different from one another. On the original Atkins® diet, for example, you eat foods high in saturated fat such as eggs, bacon, butter, and red meat. On Sugar Busters!®, you cut out white flour, sugar and starchy vegetables, but can eat high-fat fare such as butter. On the South Beach Diet™, you eat lean proteins and cut out all carbs during the first phase and then slowly step up your carb intake in phase two.

All of these diets are based on the idea that when you reduce your carbs you will reduce the hormone insulin, coaxing the body to rely on fat stores for energy. While on the surface this may seem logical and doable, it is fraught with unseen dangers to your health. Such diets do work—initially. Once you give up a food group, you generally consume fewer calories, which does result in weight loss. If 60 percent of your diet is made up of carbs and you give them all up—you just cut 60 percent of your calories. Cut that out and your weight will plummet. There no doubt about it. And promoters of low-carb diets would have you believe that the reason Americans are overweight is due to the intake of too many carbs. In reality, the reason so many Americans are overweight is due simply to the intake of too many calories.

Indeed, a review of studies done on low-carbohydrate diets that was published in the British medical journal, *The Lancet*, found that low-carb diets do result in weight loss, but not in the way low-carb diet promoters want you to think. Rather than normalizing insulin levels and forcing your body to burn fat, the diets result in weight loss because of calorie restriction and water loss.

More important, the weight you lose doesn't stay off for long. Many of my clients who have tried various low-carb diets told me they lost weight at first, but soon hit a plateau, and eventually gained it all back and more. Why? **Here's the big secret:** *Up to 25 percent of the weight lost on low-carb diets comes from your lean muscle tissue.* Why is muscle loss so strongly linked to weight gain? It is critical that you remember that lean muscles are what make up your metabolism. One pound of muscle burns up to 50 calories a day. If you lose 4 pounds on a low-carb diet, one of those pounds comes from lean muscle tissue. You'll immediately burn 50 fewer calories a day and 18,250 fewer calories a year. One pound of fat equals 3,500 calories, which equates to a five-pound fat gain in a year. And that's if you don't binge and eat even more! End result: You regain more than you lose on low-carb diets. If you lose 5 pounds of lean muscle, you will gain 26 pounds of new fat.

Let's take a closer look at the three ways low-carb diets specifically cause you to cannibalize lean muscle.

A) Stored blood sugar (glycogen) loss

You may wonder why you have a "sweet tooth." You may think, "If sugar and other sweet foods are so bad for me, why do I crave them so much?" That's a really good question, and one that should cause you to question low-carb diets even more.

To understand how cutting carbs depletes the blood sugar stored in your

Two Words to Know:

Glucose = unstored blood sugar in blood stream
Glycogen = stored blood sugar in muscles

muscles, you must take a journey back in time—to the days when men and women survived by hunting and gathering. Sure, these ancient men and women didn't have cookies and cake to feed themselves. But they did learn that sweet foods—berries, fruit, and so on—were packed with nutrients they needed for optimum energy. These foods contained carbs that went straight to their muscles, where they were stored as blood sugar called *glycogen*. When these ancient hunters and gatherers needed to move quickly—chasing down a wild animal or running away from one—their muscles could easily access these carbs and burn them for energy. Sweet foods helped our ancient ancestors to survive. That's why we evolved to love sweet tastes.

Fast forward to today. Your muscles still store the carbs you eat in the form of glycogen. When you eat carbs—say, a piece of bread—your stomach and intestines break them down into their simplest components, converting them into a form of sugar called *glucose* that then enters your bloodstream. This glucose gets shuttled into various cells in your body and is either used immediately to fuel cell reactions—such as brain function—or is stored in your muscles and liver to be used later, when needed.

You only have so much glucose floating around in your bloodstream. Whenever you use it all up, your body begins to release the glycogen stored in your muscles into a fuel it can burn for energy. Indeed, your body's favorite source of energy comes from carbohydrates. Your body can use this fuel more quickly and easily than fat or protein. Stored right there in your muscles, your body can easily convert glycogen to fuel and the energy you need to get out of bed, walk to the office, and generally fuel every task you complete all day long.

You have a reserve of glycogen stored in your muscles which can be tapped for energy and quickly burned as well. Your body has enough stored glycogen to power about ninety minutes of exercise. So you can see, you don't have much to begin with—and cutting carbs means that your gas tank will soon be empty. End result: your muscles start to shrink, and when they shrink so will your metabolism.

PHYLLIS McCLANAHAN— LOST 65 POUNDS

Name: Phyllis McClanahan
Height: 5'3"
Age: 56
Starting weight: 252 lbs.
Current weight: 187 lbs.
Other: Full-time career woman;
  grandmother of 3

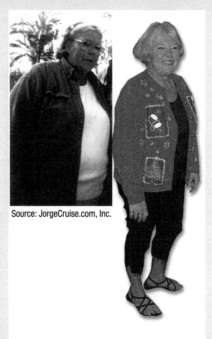

Source: JorgeCruise.com, Inc.

"Before I started the 3-Hour Diet™ I was pretty much okay with myself, even though I knew that weight was always a problem. It didn't seem to affect my ability to do much. I was active in sports, never had a problem getting a job, and always had a fun social life.

"I was never that concerned because anytime I wanted I could lose 30 or 40 pounds I'd try to eliminate carbs from my diet. I could lose what I wanted in three or four months. Then I would gradually gain it all back, plus a few more. I didn't really get it. I didn't care if the diet was healthy. I just wanted to lose the weight. I yo-yo'd all my life.

"Now I get it. It is about a lifestyle change. I still do what I want now and eat what I want, but I have learned the nutritional value associated with it. Instead of depriving myself of things I like, I just eat them in moderation. And that's easy because I get to eat every three hours. The best thing about the diet is when I get off track a little (which sometimes happens), I don't gain. I don't have to go back and start over again. **This is the first time in my life that I have kept 65 pounds off.** I still have a ways to go, but I really get it now thanks to Jorge."

Phyllis's Secrets to Success

> ➤ Put your meals in your computer scheduler so it will beep and remind you to eat.
> ➤ Know that being healthy is your choice. Do it for you.

B) Water loss

The second way low-carb diets cause you to lose muscle is from water loss. Glycogen depletion leads to water loss. Every gram of glycogen in muscles is stored with three grams of water. When blood sugar is low, the body pulls glycogen out of the muscles, which releases the water, causing easy weight loss on the scale. Keep in mind that you are losing water.

Another way you lose water from your lean muscles on a low-carb diet is by burning body fat. Yes, on low-carb diets you do burn body fat, particularly in the beginning. But when your body burns fat in the absence of carbohydrates, the fat is only partially broken down, which creates by-products called *ketones*. Usually your body removes these by-products very efficiently, but when you burn too much fat and too little (or no) carbohydrate, ketones begin to build up, sometimes to extremely dangerous levels. This condition is called ketosis. In Dr. Robert Atkins's diet books, he called ketosis a "wonderful process" because, after all, you are forcing your body to burn fat for fuel. Unfortunately this wonderful process has a toxic effect. When your body burns too much fat and no carbohydrate for energy, nitrogen is also released. And nitrogen is toxic in the body. Bottom line: ketosis places your body into a toxic state that alters the acid-alkaline balance in your blood and the rest of your body. It can cause everything from dizziness, fatigue, bad breath, hair loss, and even death if it goes on long enough.

Fortunately your body does not want you to die—so it instinctively and automatically instructs the flushing of those toxins out with your body's reserves of stored water. Many dieters think this is a good thing. They spend two weeks on a low-carb diet and see their weight plummet on the scale. It's not unusual to lose 6, 7 or more pounds during the first week on one of these diets. Yet it's important to know that while this may seem like stunning weight loss, the weight doesn't come from where you want it—your fat stores—it comes from where you don't want to lose it: your muscles. The end result is that your muscles shrink even further.

C) Fatigue and depression lead to a sedentary lifestyle.

Ok, so now you've depleted blood sugar and water from your bloodstream and muscles. Your body is starting to hit the wall. Your metabolism is already grinding to a halt. Now you're feeling so tired—not to mention cranky and depressed—that you're going to burn even fewer calories simply from sitting on your butt more often.

One Other Way You Lose Muscle

Although your brain prefers to use glucose for fuel (to the tune of 150 grams per day) it can make an exception and use ketones for about 50 percent of its energy needs. But the other half *must* come from glucose. The problem is that if you have dramatically lowered your carb intake, you leave your body no choice but to create glucose from your muscle protein fiber. They are the actual protein fibers that create the structural support of your cells and muscles. And now these fibers are broken down, causing even further damage to your muscles and metabolism.

Why is this so? Ask any serious athlete or coach and you'll find out about the importance of carbohydrates for quick and long-lasting energy. As Australian exercise physiologist Mark Hargreaves wrote in the *Journal of Sport Science*, "increased dietary carbohydrate intake in the days before competition increases muscle glycogen levels and enhances exercise performance." Serious runners, cyclists and other endurance athletes would never think of trying a low-carb diet. They know all too well that carbs equal energy.

You don't need to be a runner or cyclist to experience a drop in energy with a low-carb diet. Yep, ask anyone who has done a low-carb diet long term and they will tell you that they are constantly fatigued or depressed. Why? Carbs and sugars are your brain's preferred sources for energy. When your brain runs low on this important fuel, you'll begin to feel muddled. You won't be able to think clearly. You'll get a headache. Your mood will plummet. You'll feel very tired just doing simple everyday things: walking from your car to the grocery store, climbing a flight of steps, or carrying laundry out to the clothes line. And you'll start craving the very foods you are trying not to eat: carbs.

An online client of mine, Dona Buth, says, "I was on the Atkins® diet about 5 years ago. I followed it for two weeks. I definitely had less energy. It was not the right diet for me. I just couldn't eat that way. It was not a healthy diet for me." Another one of my clients, Karen Rudolph, put it this way, "When I first began the Atkins® diet, I had wonderful amounts of energy, but as the diet progressed, I had less energy—and that side effect took the greatest toll on me. I became a little confused and a little less focused, and even short-tempered. The most frustrating part was that I followed the diet precisely for two and a half months. Initially I lost 11 pounds, which was great. But then slowly but surely I began to gain weight back even though I was following the diet perfectly."

Researchers have documented very clearly that low-carb diets lead to fatigue. In a study conducted at Southern Illinois University and published in the journal *Perception and Motor Skills,* seventeen participants who tried a low-carb diet for three weeks rated their fatigue levels as higher than before they tried the low-carb diet.

Think about it. When you are fatigued do you feel like exercising or moving? No way. Instead you'll circle the parking lot five or more times, waiting to find the spot closest to the grocery store door. You'll toss your clothes into the dryer rather than hang them out on the line. Instead of going for a walk, you'll lie on the couch and watch re-runs. You know the drill. If you can save some effort, you will.

All of these little decisions about how much to move—or not move— make a big difference in terms of your overall calorie burn. A number of years ago, researchers found that fidgeting—those tiny movements like shaking your foot or tapping your finger—can burn about 75 or more extra calories a day. Researchers also have documented that our sedentary lifestyles composed of power car windows, elevators, moving walkways, and E-Z Pass cause us to burn 250 fewer calories a day than we did twenty years ago. That lack of calorie burning adds up quickly. The only way to maintain your weight is to eat even fewer calories. Eventually, something has to give. You break the diet and gain back the weight.

And guess what? This lack of movement due to fatigue has long-term consequences. That old adage of "use it or lose it" is absolutely true when it comes down to your lean muscle tissue. That's why I originally wrote my *8 Minutes in the Morning*® books to get people to strength train and tone their muscles. In just eight minutes a day, they could create the muscle tissue needed to rev up their metabolic furnace.

One of the golden rules about muscle is this: Use it or lose it. As you move less and less due to fatigue caused by a low-carb diet, your muscle tissue will begin to shrink, and your metabolism will slow down even more.

Point 2: How low-carb diets cause you to gain more weight

Marketing misunderstandings

Remember the low-fat craze? Ten years ago, as Americans cut fat in order to slim down and improve their health, food manufacturers came out with more than 3,000 new low-fat food products. In the decade that followed, however, Americans got even fatter and more unhealthy. The number of overweight people jumped by 15 percent. What happened? Low-fat products were far from low-calorie. In order to preserve optimal taste, food manufacturers replaced the fat with sugar, so the overall calorie content was roughly the same. At the same time, Americans dished up larger servings—and our waistlines expanded.

Today, the same applies to low-carb products. More than 2,000 new low-carb products have hit the supermarket shelves, ranging from brownie mixes to pasta to bread. And here's the bottom line: many of these products contain the same number of calories as the regular carb versions—or more. The "low-carb" chicken wings at T.G.I. Friday's® contain the same number of calories (more than 1,000 for 24 wings) as the original version. The Powerbar Pria® Carb Select™ has 180 calories, compared to 110 calories in the regular bar. Manufacturers have reduced the carb content of many other products simply by reducing the serving size. For example, Thomas's low-carb bagels contain 140 calories and 23 grams of carbs, compared to the company's multigrain bagels' 300 calories and 57 grams of carbs—but they are half the size.

In addition, some so-called low-carb products aren't even low in carbs. The Pure De-lite™ chocolate bar, for example, claims to be low-carb but actually contains 20 grams of total carbohydrates. This has led to many low-carb dieters eating more carbs and calories than they think. For three years, a market research company called the NPD Group examined the food records of 11,000 people on low-carb diets. The 5 percent of people who ate the fewest carbs actually consumed an average 128 grams of carbs a day, still much more than the 20 to 60 grams that most low-carb diets recommend.

As with the low-fat craze, it doesn't do your waistline or hips and thighs any good if you consume the same number of calories or more than before. If you gobble up low-carb products with wild abandon—and end up consuming more calories as a result—you're going to gain weight. It's that simple.

The "great carb tradeoff"

When the low-fat lifestyle was all the rage, food manufacturers found many interesting ways to replace the fat in various formerly "fatty foods." You may remember olestra, the fake fat that turned out to cause anal leakages, among other problems. One other popular replacement was hydrogenated

LOW-CARB PRODUCTS VS. REGULAR PRODUCTS

Think low-carb means low-calorie? Think again. Some low-carb products contain the same number or more calories than their "regular" counterparts. Read the labels.

ITEM DESCRIPTION	LOW-CARB PORTION & # OF CALORIES	REGULAR PORTION & # OF CALORIES
Atkins® Pepperoni Pizza (6.1 oz) vs. Celeste® Regular Pepperoni Pizza (5.58 oz)	Serves 1 = 440	Serves 1 = 410
Anthony's Reduced Carb Elbow Macaroni vs. Barilla® Regular Elbow Macaroni	½ cup = 200	½ cup = 200
Ragu® Carb Options Hearty Italian Style Sauce w/sausage vs. Ragu® Rich and Meaty Classic Italian Sauce w/ sausage and beef	½ cup = 160	½ cup = 130
Carb Option Decaf Lemon Flavored Iced Tea Mix vs. any regular brand of the same	0	0
Post® Carb Well Cinnamon Crunch cereal vs. Life® Cinnamon cereal (Quaker®)	½ cup = 110	½ cup = 80

fat, the same fat found in margarine. We now know that this fat is more harmful to our health than saturated fat, the type of fat found in animal products.

The same is now true with low-carb products. To remove the carbs, food manufacturers must put something else back in. They use all sorts of replacements, including soy flour, almond flour, the sugar substitute Splenda®, and sugar alcohols. The jury is still out on the safety of many of these replacements. Sugar alcohols, for example, may actually raise blood sugar levels. They also have been linked to flatulence and diarrhea. And although soy is generally considered a healthful food, too much of it can cause problems because it contains phytoestrogens that mimic the hormone estrogen in the body and can contribute to certain causes of breast cancer in women. Too much soy has also been linked to poor brain function and the formation of kidney stones.

About 25 grams of soy protein a day is good for you, but if you gobble up one low-carb product after another, you're eating much more than that—too much.

What Are "Net Carbs"?

Back in 2001 Atkins® Nutritionals, Inc. created this term, and now plenty of other low-carb companies have followed suit. It supposedly means how many carbs there are in foods after you remove the fiber content. Yet the Food and Drug Administration has no official definition for it. According to the Food and Drug Administration, there's no such thing as net carbs. And "net carbs" are not required to be listed on food labels. Carbs are carbs.

Others, including myself, believe this net carbs stuff is all nonsense. Food manufacturers are simply replacing sugar and starch with sugar alcohols, sweeteners made with hydrogenated starch molecules. Just like regular sugar, sugar alcohols contain calories, ranging from 0.2 to 3.0 calories per gram. Carbs are carbs and calories are calories. By getting you to focus on these so-called net carbs, food manufacturers are distracting you from the real truth: how many calories a food contains. In the end, it's the calories that matter. If you really want to know how many carbs are in a food, ignore the "net carbs" label and instead look at the numbers of "total carbohydrate," a nutrition fact that *is* policed by the FDA. Don't be surprised if the two numbers are wildly different!

And here is some news that might surprise you even more. As of October 2004, the same company that invented the term "net carbs," Atkins® Nutritionals, Inc, has now officially dropped the term from its food labeling, calling it "imprecise." This move came just months before the FDA was expected to issue new food-labeling guidelines for carbohydrate content.

Binge eating

Low-carb diets can also cause depression and mood swings that can lead to emotional binge eating. Indeed, *Self*® magazine recently dubbed the problem "the Atkins Attitude," defining it as "a biological (and attitudinal) response to a chronically low-carb diet, which is characterized by grouchiness (I'm hungry), distractability (Did you say pasta?), even depression (I miss you, french fries.)"

Research indicates that low-carbohydrate diets promote depression by lowering levels of the neurotransmitter serotonin in the brain. In research conducted by Judith Wurtman, PhD, at the Massachusetts Institute of Technology, rats fed a low-carbohydrate diet for three weeks had lower levels of serotonin than rats fed a normal diet. Additional research completed at MIT found lower levels of serotonin in women on the Atkins diet.

Serotonin influences your mood and your appetite. Low serotonin levels are thought to cause depression, anger, and hunger. Your brain needs carbs to manufacture levels of this chemical, but when you are on a low-carb diet, you're consistently low on blood sugar—the brain's main fuel source. The brain can also, in a pinch, burn fat for fuel, but this creates by-products that lower serotonin levels even more. Women may be particularly at risk for depression and mood swings on low-carb diets because they produce less serotonin than men. *First for Women* magazine has reported receiving hundreds of letters from frustrated women on low-carb diets. When deprived of serotonin, women are biologically programmed to crave foods (carbohydrates) that boost its production. In addition to serotonin, you also need carbs for your body to produce the brain chemical dopamine, which combats energy slumps and generally keeps you feeling good.

Some research shows that low-carb diets cause a response in the body similar to people undergoing long-term stress. When you restrict carbs, the body releases the stress hormone cortisol, which promotes belly fat. This hormone turns down fat burning and increases carb burning. It also increases mood swings and emotional stress, which causes more cortisol to be released.

And that's the problem with mood swings: not only do they make you feel crummy, but they also make you more likely to overeat. If you tend to reward yourself with comfort foods to begin with, a low-carb diet is only going to strengthen that tendency. This is why low-carb diets often end in a binge. Your mood plummets and eventually you give in, stuffing yourself with bread, pasta, and any and all other starches you can get your hands on. Once you break the diet, the weight gain begins.

Indeed, a recent review in the *Journal of the American College of Cardiology* found that few people can stick with a low-carb diet long enough to achieve results. Between 20 and 43 percent of people who start low-carb diets end up bingeing and cheating—and quitting the diet—long before the "diet" is officially over.

Point 3: Additional health risks with low-carb diets

It doesn't do much good to lose weight if you destroy your health in the process. That was the belief of a 53-year-old Florida man who sued the Atkins® company because he says the diet raised his cholesterol, which clogged his arteries so much that he needed surgery to open them. After just two months on the diet, his cholesterol jumped from 146 to 230 milligrams per deciliter.

Here are just some of the adverse health reactions that more than 3,500 studies have linked to low-carb diets:

Digestive woes. Because most low-carb diets are also low in fiber, they tend to cause constipation. In a study completed at Duke University, 68 percent of low-carb dieters suffered from constipation—compared to only 35 percent of those on a regular diet. An additional 23 percent suffered from diarrhea, which ironically can also be caused by lack of fiber. Fiber is found in plant foods such as fruits, vegetables, legumes, and whole grains—most of which are no-no's on low-carb diets.

Kidney problems. Research conducted at Harvard University shows low-carb diets speed the loss of kidney function in people who are already sick. High blood pressure and diabetes are also risk factors for kidney disease, so you should stay away from low-carb diets if you have one of those conditions. High protein, low-carb diets cause the body to excrete more calcium through the urine, which has been shown to increase the risk of kidney stones.

Heart disease. This is the top killer of both men and women. Research conducted at the Fleming Heart and Health Institute in Omaha, Nebraska, shows that the high fat content of some low-carb diets raises levels of blood fats, which causes the inner linings of arteries to become inflamed. According to this research, blood flow to the heart decreased by 40 percent after people spent a year on the Atkins® diet, whereas blood flow increased by 40 percent in people who followed a low-fat, high carbohydrate diet. Although other studies contradict these findings—showing that the Atkins® diet promotes heart health—these studies included consumption of nutritional supplements such as fish oil, which may have counteracted the detrimental effects of the diet.

A shorter lifespan. Low-carb diets tend to be low in a number of important nutrients, including vitamins E, A, thiamin, B_6, and folate; minerals calcium, zinc, magnesium, and potassium; and fiber. Research conducted at Harvard University on 60,000 nurses shows that diets high in fruits, vegetables, and whole grains—the very foods you shun on a low-carb diet—led to a longer life than the diets' of women who ate fewer of those foods.

Weak bones. Low-carb diets cause the body to excrete calcium in the urine, pulling it out of the bones. Studies show calcium loss on low-carb diets is 65 percent above normal rates.

Bad breath. Excess protein in the diet creates a surplus of acid in the digestive system. This allows yeast and bacteria to flourish, opening valves in the digestive system and allowing these bugs to create bad breath. Burning fat for energy also creates by-products (called ketones, mentioned earlier) which are released through the breath and the urine, making both smell foul.

Lessened fertility. According to research performed on mice and presented at a fertility conference, low-carb diets may hinder a woman's chances of conceiving. The culprit may be high levels of ammonium in the blood, which can adversely affect embryo growth and development. This could cause a fetus to spontaneously abort.

Gout. When the body is unable to get rid of excess waste products from the excessive consumption of fat and protein, gout occurs. This is a painful swelling of the joints resulting from a build-up of waste in the blood. Due to dehydration and stress, the kidneys are unable to accommodate its release.

Hair loss. One of the things we learned from firsthand feedback from our clients is that while on a low-carb diet, many of them experienced hair loss, even within the first few weeks. Many clients who had experienced this were emotionally devastated, which lead to depression and a lowered self-image. They felt less attractive and, in some extreme cases, were even forced to incorporate hairpieces and full wigs into their daily dress.

There's yet another reason why low-carb diets may make you fat. In addition to all of these health consequences, low-carb diets can hit you in another place that hurts: your wallet. You can't sustain them because they are expensive. According to *USA Today*,® strict adherence to the Atkins® diet costs about three times more for the food than regular, non-low-carb items.

I hope you can see that low-carb diets are not the way to go. While they may help you lose weight in the short term, the long term is what matters. Losing weight on a low-carb diet is like winning the lottery one day, only to have to pay it all back with interest six months later. Don't you want to win the lottery and keep your loot long-term?

Then make a promise to yourself to stop the deprivation and bring back carbs in your life. I will show you how in this book. By bringing back the carbs you will stop damaging your metabolism, end the carb-rage that leads to binge eating, avoid major health dangers, and most importantly, bring back the joy of eating!

Use the information I've provided you here to make this all-important decision not only for yourself, but also for your loved ones. You can help loved ones make better choices about their health and, more important, end the yo-yo dieting cycle once and for all!

THREE

WHY OTHER FAD DIETS MAKE YOU FAT

Before the 3-Hour Diet™, I could not stand looking in the mirror, buying clothes or even going out into the world. I made a joke about the fact that the person I saw in the mirror was some other person I did not know. My husband joked that he could no longer afford to feed me out in restaurants. Whether it was the Beverly Hills Diet or the potato diet, you name it, I've tried it. Now thanks to Jorge Cruise, I am eating my way thin. My body has responded to this by dropping 35 pounds in only twelve weeks. I'm totally amazed that this works, and I am optimistic about the future. I have gone from a size 16 to a 8, and I have done it without any exercise. Now I look in the mirror and I am beginning to see the person I used to be. I will be forever grateful to Jorge for giving me my life back."

—BRANDY TROCHE—LOST 50 POUNDS

There are many other fad diets that will end up making you fat, besides low-carb diets. Yep, many of my clients at JorgeCruise.com have shared with me how they have only done shakes, stopped eating fat, or eaten soup—and only soup—for weeks on end. They've skipped meals, survived on popcorn, and generally tried to starve off the fat.

Such extreme methods, however, always backfire. Fad diets never work.

It is critical that you realize that fad diets—including low-carb diets— almost always result in failure. They do this because they always require you to remove something from your diet. They ask you to deprive yourself of something that you like or love. Think about it . . . how many times have you given up X, Y, or Z? By depriving yourself of foods you enjoy, you will sabotage your success. You will binge and it will be over.

My goal for you in this chapter is very simple. It's to get you to clearly see why you must never again eat a diet that restricts your food options or tells you to remove something. It's time to end *all* deprivation. Think of this chapter as your final step before you enter the 3-Hour Diet™ revolution.

Just imagine enjoying all the foods you like to eat, without eliminating any food groups ever again. Perhaps even more important, after reading this chapter, you will feel 100 percent confident about your road to weight-loss success. You'll turn on a light bulb that will illuminate your first steps toward your goal.

The Fads

Let's take a close look at the history of fad diets—and there have been lots of them over the years. I want you to see just how silly and unhealthy most of these diets really are, and how they result in weight-loss failure. Once you see the truth you will be set free.

The first fad diet dates back to 1087, when William the Conqueror took to his bed and consumed nothing but alcohol to help himself lose weight. In the 1600s, the dairy diet was in vogue, as its followers believed drinking copious amounts would keep them slender. In the 1800s Lord Byron swore that vinegar could result in weight loss.

And the fads went on and on. Thousands of fad diets have been created, but the sad news is that not one of them has made a permanent, positive change. If they worked, we'd all be skinny, and we're not. Look at the chart on the next page to see what many of these diets tell you to give up—and why they are dangerous to your health. Then read on to take a closer look at some of these diets.

Let's take a closer look at some of these diets.

DIET	WHAT'S REMOVED	WHY IT'S DANGEROUS
Atkins®, South Beach™ (low-carb)	CARBOHYDRATES!!!	Your body must have carbs and fiber to survive. Going on a low-carb diet will result in losing up to 25 percent of your lean muscle mass. See chapter 2 for all the details.
Hollywood 48-Hour Miracle®	ALL FOOD for 2 days	When you fast on juice for 48 hours, you place your body in deep starvation mode. This causes you to lose up to 50 percent of your lean muscle mass, eroding your metabolism as a result.
Cabbage Soup	Most foods	This super-low calorie diet will not only lead to cravings (cabbage soup just doesn't quite have the mouth appeal of a small piece of pie), but also lowers your metabolism as your body consumes its muscle tissue.
Grapefruit	Most foods	There are no miracle foods, not even grapefruit! This is a super-low-calorie diet that will cause your body to consume its lean muscle tissue, destroying your metabolism.
Fat-free diets	Flavor	Fat makes food taste good. It also helps slow digestion, making you feel satisfied. Cutting all of the fat from your meals will only result in bingeing later on.
Blood Type Diet	Freedom	When you adhere to a detailed list of foods, you lose the ability to eat the foods you want, when you want them. This leads to cravings and binges, and future weight gain.
Popcorn	Most of your snacks	On this diet you snack on popcorn. But this snack food can actually contain more calories than potato chips. Besides, eating the same snack every day gets boring, and you eventually drop off the diet.
Raw Food	Satisfaction	Warm food smells and tastes good. Eating only raw foods is not only time-consuming, it's also boring. You'll soon break the diet and regain the weight.
Peanut Butter Diet/ Ice Cream Diet	Variety	On these diets, you indulge in either peanut butter or ice cream every single day—in addition to an otherwise healthful assortment of foods. What if you want a chocolate bar or some other dessert? You'll break the diet and gain back the weight.

The Hollywood 48-Hour Miracle Diet®

This "cleansing" diet can cause you to lose a large amount of weight within a very short period of time—forty-eight hours. During the diet, you drink a blend of fruit juices but eat no solid food. The fruit juice blend acts as a natural laxative, flushing out your system. The typical person has 3 to 10 pounds of waste matter (feces) in their intestines. This is where a large part of the weight loss on the Miracle diet comes from. Within forty-eight hours, you lose between 2 and 5 pounds of waste matter. The rest of the weight loss generally comes from water loss, because the diet acts as a diuretic. You can lose anywhere from 1 to 6 pounds of water over forty-eight hours. Overall, you may lose up to 1 pound of fat and up to 2 pounds of muscle tissue.

It's no wonder the weight comes back quickly. Losing 1 to 2 pounds of muscle lowers your metabolism, which means you must eat 50 to 100 fewer calories every day to prevent that pound of fat from creeping back on your frame. Plus, if you resume your old, low fiber eating habits, the fecal matter will also build back up. You end up at the same weight as you started—or worse, heavier!

The Grapefruit Diet

This diet promises to help you shed 52 pounds in two and a half months. That's an average of 5 pounds a week. To stick to the diet, you must follow a set meal plan that not only includes lots of grapefruit (supposedly for fat burning), but also a little protein—and not much else. A typical breakfast is half a grapefruit. A typical lunch includes half a grapefruit, an egg, a piece of toast, and some salad. A typical dinner includes half a grapefruit, half a head of lettuce with sliced tomato, and two eggs. Are you hungry yet? I sure am.

The diet's proponents claim it's the combination of foods that burn the fat, but the truth is that no one food will magically burn off the fat. You lose weight on the grapefruit diet for the same reason you lose weight on any fad diet. By carefully adhering to a set food plan and giving up a number of foods, you'll be consuming *fewer calories*. Once you begin to eat normally, however, the weight will come back, as anyone who has tried the grapefruit diet knows.

The Cabbage Soup Diet

This diet promises that you can lose 10 pounds in seven days. On this diet, you can eat as much cabbage soup as you want, whenever you want. You make the soup with a head of cabbage, some onions, peppers, diced tomatoes, celery, and onion soup mix. Because the soup is mostly water and watery vegetables, it contains very few calories.

In addition to the soup, you are allowed to eat an odd assortment of foods on various days. On the first day of the diet, you may eat all the fruit you want—except bananas—and cabbage soup. On the second day you can eat as many vegetables as you want, and cabbage soup. On another day you can eat as many bananas and drink as much skim milk as you want—along with cabbage soup—but nothing else. This goes on for seven days.

This diet helps you shed pounds for two reasons. First, most of the foods you are allowed to eat are low in calories. Second, you are only allowed to eat a few foods on any given day. Such food boredom leads to undereating. In the end, you do lose weight. Again, you can't keep this type of eating plan up forever. No one can survive on fruit one day, vegetables the next, and bananas the next. It's just not feasible. As with all fad diets, once you break the diet, the weight creeps back.

Fat-Free Diets

Popular in the 1980s and '90s, these diets claimed you could lose weight by cutting the fat. Many people did lose weight as they switched from a diet rich in fatty meats and cheeses to one rich in whole grains, fruits, and vegetables. But many other people didn't. They switched from a similarly fatty diet to one rich in commercially prepared low-fat foods such as fat-free ice cream, pretzels, and margarine. What they didn't bargain for was that many of the low- and no-fat products contained just as many calories as—if not more than—their higher fat cousins.

Many of the people who successfully lost weight on fat-free diets eventually gained it back. It's just not feasible to keep your fat intake so low for so long. Fat does have a purpose: It makes foods taste delicious, and even has many important functions in the human body. Cut fat intake too low and you get food cravings, mood swings, even depression. Once you start bingeing on high-fat foods, the weight comes back.

Height: 5'3½"
Age: 32
Starting weight: 245 lbs.
Current weight: 190 lbs.
Other: Married with one child,
    work-at-home artist

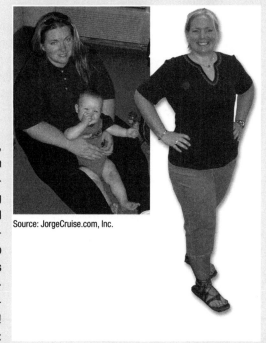

Source: JorgeCruise.com, Inc.

"Before Jorge's 3-Hour Diet™, I had become disgusted with myself. My health was declining, my body was aging prematurely and sagging, and my energy level was nonexistent. I didn't want my son to grow up embarrassed of his overweight mom! More important, I wanted to be able to enjoy an active lifestyle with him!

"I have tried many diets: low-fat, no-fat, low-carb, excessive exercise. None was easy and they all failed me in the long run. Most made me feel like a failure for not being able to follow the strict regimen, so I would give up.

"Since beginning the 3-Hour Diet™, **I've noticed a huge increase in energy. I have the stamina to make it through the day without needing a nap.** With this increased energy, my activity level has dramatically gone up! I now love to get out and hike or swim. Even better are the changes in my body! My knees and elbows have reappeared. My sagging areas are tightening up. I am excited each week by the new contours developing as the fat is replaced with lean muscle!

"The best part of all is that I never feel deprived. This is why it works for me as a lifestyle! No food is off-limits! Each evening I treat myself to a Hershey® miniature chocolate! Because I eat every 3 hours, I never feel starved. Since I have learned how to feed my body properly, my body rewards me with the energy to be active, which in turn, burns fat and builds muscle. I am no longer a dieting failure! I'm on my way to a healthy beautiful body for the rest of my life."

Michelle's Secrets to Success

➤ Get a watch with five alarms set to go off so you never miss a snack or meal.
➤ Prepare all your menus for the week and go grocery shopping on Sunday.
➤ Divide your snacks out into proper servings in zip-locks and always keep a few in the diaper bag or purse so you are never caught without a snack!
➤ Steam lots of veggies. That way you always have leftovers and no excuse for not eating veggies!

The Blood Type Diet

In this series of books, you follow a diet based on your blood type. The promise is that you'll improve digestion and therefore lose weight. Each diet is extreme and difficult to adhere to. You must adhere to a very detailed list of foods that you can and cannot eat. For example, Type Os are supposed to eat lots of meat and absolutely no wheat, whereas Type As are supposed to follow a strict vegetarian diet. None of the diets is easy to maintain, and the benefits for maintaining any of the diets are speculative at best.

The Raw Food Diet

On this diet you eat only raw foods. Promoters claim that raw foods contain certain enzymes that are better for your weight and health. The way you really lose weight on this diet, however, is through calorie deprivation. It can take twenty-four hours or longer to "cook" your raw food meals in a dehydrator. When it takes that long to prepare a meal, you're going to end up skipping meals, pure and simple.

Here's another problem. How long do you think you can stick with a raw food diet? During the winter, won't you miss a bowl of warm soup or some fresh warm bread straight from the oven? Sure you will. Once you break the diet, you'll regain the weight.

Now I do want to say something good about raw foods. When my father was diagnosed with prostate cancer, he and I attended a wonderful health center in San Diego that prescribed raw foods only. The reason he went was to truly cleanse his body and try to overcome cancer, not lose weight. If you have a family member that has a serious health challenge,

What Is a Fad Diet?

It's a fad diet if it . . .

Promises fast weight loss every week (more than what doctors recommend as safe: 2 pounds a week)

Eliminates certain foods or food groups

Drastically slashes your calories (below 1200 calories)

Doesn't include the medically sound information explaining why it works

Encourages the purchase of commercial products as the only way to follow it

Includes a "magical" food

then check out their website: www.optimumhealth.org—it might help save their life. It did with my dad.

Why Deprivation Equals Failure

Just about all fad diets have one thing in common: they make you forego certain foods. Any diet that bans certain foods from the menu is a deprivation diet. Let's take a closer look at how and why deprivation leads to bingeing.

Think about it. Giving up bread for eight weeks may sound doable, but how about a year? How about the rest of your life? Humans are hardwired to crave a variety of foods. If you stop eating carbohydrates or proteins or fats, your body will eventually crave those foods more than ever. Then when you give in and reintroduce those foods to your diet, you binge and gorge, eating huge amounts that you would have never eaten had you not been on the deprivation diet in the first place.

I hear about this problem over and over again from my millions of on-line clients at JorgeCruise.com. Before they could lose weight and keep it off, they all had to learn that deprivation usually causes more weight gain in the long term. Research shows that merely thinking about banning foods from your diet can bring on food cravings. A study done at the University of Toronto found that students who were told that they were about to embark on a week-long diet that restricted particular foods were more likely to consume more food the night before the diet than other students who were not told they would soon start a diet. A different study done at the University of Florida in Gainesville found that students who routinely deprived themselves of certain foods responded to pictures of certain foods with increased heart rates and more sensitive startle reflexes. Finally, another study done at Louisiana State University found that people with the most flexible eating habits were more likely to eat reasonable food portions than those with the most restrained eating habits.

Fad diets almost always end with a binge. Scientists have shown that rats and other animals will respond to calorie restriction by binge eating. Other research shows that as soon as people begin a fad diet, they become preoccupied with food. It's even more important to avoid fad diets if you have binge eating disorder, a diagnosed condition that affects millions of Americans. People with this disorder eat abnormally large amounts of food and feel out of control over their eating. They exhibit the following behaviors: eating more rapidly than normal, eating until uncomfortably full, eating when not physically hungry, and eating alone out of embarrassment of how much they are eating. Although the causes are unknown, many experts believe dieting can make the condition worse by triggering depression, which, in turn, triggers the disorder.

Bring Back the Freedom and Joy of Eating

So if not a fad diet, then what? How can you lose weight if you don't restrict your eating? That's what the 3-Hour Diet™ is all about.

On the 3-Hour Diet™, you will learn how to eat without restricting food options, ever! By not restricting the options you eat, you will put an end to cravings and bingeing. You will experience a new freedom each time you enjoy a meal.

There are no banned foods on the 3-Hour Diet™. That's right: not one banned food. You can eat bread and cake and butter.

As Laura Porter, one of my clients put it, "When I tried fad diets, the desire for goodies was painful. I would usually end the diet because eventually I would give into cravings and would just go back to junk food. Something unusual has happened with the 3-Hour Diet™, however. I am not having cravings. I am convinced that it is because I eat every three hours. When I eat it is all I can do to get the amount of food that I have to have on the plan. I am so full that I do not want to snack. My desire to snack is gone. I feel like I finally have found a diet that is right for me."

I know it's not easy to walk away from the world of fad diets. The promise of quick and easy weight loss is very alluring and sometimes very convincing.

I challenge you to make a commitment to yourself today. Promise yourself that you will start a new approach for the next twenty-eight days. The 3-Hour Diet™ will help you shed 2 pounds every week and that amount is perfect since much more would lead to saggy skin that would not recoil as the weight came off.

So get ready to join the revolution!

PART II

How It Works —Visual Timing™

FOUR

HOW TO SUCCESSFULLY
DO THE 3-HOUR DIET™

oday, when I look in the mirror, I see a healthy,
active person. My knees don't hurt like they did
seven weeks ago. I really do feel healthier now.
This is a big change for me—a change for the
better. I want to enjoy my retirement. I thank
Jorge for my success. I am now on the right path
for an active lifestyle."

—DONA BUTH—LOST 20 POUNDS

Most of us pay close attention to the clock. We set an alarm to wake us in
time for work. We strive to leave work by a particular time in order to beat
rush-hour traffic. We structure our lives around the time we need to pick
the kids up from day care, soccer practice, and play dates.

Yet too many of us seem to get out of sync when it comes to eating.
Rather than having an eating schedule, many people tend to eat only when
it occurs to them. They rush out the door in the morning, forgetting to eat
breakfast or intentionally skipping it to save time and calories. They get
swept up at work, and realize at two or three in the afternoon that they
haven't eaten lunch—and for many people that is their first meal of the day.

They complete errands and other tasks after work, only remembering to eat dinner when they are too hungry to stand it.

When you eat is critical. As I mentioned in chapter 1, it's essential that you know that successfully losing weight and keeping it off is all about *timing*.

Yet most people use bad timing by eating sporadically. You eat sporadically anytime you allow more than 3 hours to pass between meals. This causes the body to switch from a fat-burning mode to a fat-preservation mode. Instead of fat, the body burns muscle tissue and your metabolism plummets as a result. This leads to fat gain.

So to get thin, you need to create a consistent eating schedule. That's the secret way to lose weight and keep it off. What exactly does this mean? You may be wondering again, "Is it just about eating every 3 hours? Is that all there is?" The answer is no. Although this program is very simple, there's a little bit more. You see, the key is that it must become *automatic* for you. Your eating schedule must become effortless and easy. It's all about learning how to use my Visual Timing™ formula.

The power of Visual Timing™ will free you from your past dieting failures. You will at last have an enjoyable and automatic way to eat everyday. Specifically, I promise that by following the 3-Hour Diet™ you will lose up to 2 pounds a week from your belly first and bring back the joy of eating!

The Power of Visual Timing™

The goal of Visual Timing™ is to make eating every 3 hours completely effortless and automatic. In this way, you will not only lose the weight, but keep it off long term. How will Visual Timing™ do this for you? Visual Timing™ involves two critical secrets.

Secret 1: The 3-Hour Timeline™

The first key is to learn *when* to eat. This involves learning *when* to start eating, *how* to keep going through the day, and *when* to stop. Chapter 5 will help you do all this, by uncovering my **3-Hour Timeline**™ system. This simple visual planner will help ensure that eating on time (what I call *cruise-time*) becomes effortless and automatic for you. In this chapter, you will learn how to create your ideal eating schedule. This is very important because you will never have to worry again about when you should eat. You will know exactly when to eat every day. Automatically your life will become simpler and your mind will have one less thing to think about. It's all about one word: simplicity. The 3-Hour Timeline™ will make sure you start eating at the right time in the morning, keep eating on time throughout the day, and stop eating at the right time at the end of the day. You will love it.

Secret 2: The 3-Hour Plate™

In chapter 6 you will also learn how to eat anything with my visual all-new **3-Hour Plate**™ system. This super-simple eating method will ensure you never again have to deprive yourself of carbohydrates, proteins, or fats. It will give you true freedom. Then, in chapters 12 and 13, you will find my all-new food lists and yummy meal ideas for breakfast, lunch and dinner. All the meals you make—whether you follow my suggestions in chapter 13 or create your own with the guidance of my 3-Hour Plate™—will be healthy and delicious. You'll eat from all of the food groups: proteins, fats, *and* carbohydrates. That's right. Carbs are *not* off-limits. Remember from chapter 2 what happens to lean muscle when you don't get enough carbohydrates? You lose up to 25 percent of your muscle mass. That will never happen again. You'll also never crave foods that are off-limits—because no foods are off-limits! Just imagine eating chocolate, bread, or fast food. You will never feel the need to cheat, sneak, or binge. Good eating will finally be yours to have!

Ensure your Success

Okay, so now I want to help motivate you to your success. This will ensure that you stay inspired to succeed. You see, sometimes we can have the best tools in front of us that could change our lives, but because we think we can't do it, we don't do it. What you must do right now is prove to yourself that you *will* achieve success with the 3-Hour Diet™.

How are new habits and ideas born? How do you become so certain that you can do it—that you *will* do it? You do so by changing your belief system about what you can and cannot do. Yep, because if you think you can, you will. And if you think you can't, you won't. If you are thinking right now that since you have failed at every other diet in the past, and odds are you will fail here too, then you have sealed your fate. You must not let that happen.

You will do this in two steps that help you break away from any negative thoughts and help you use positive thinking to meet your goals. By the time you are done with them, you will feel your confidence truly soar.

Height: 5' 7"
Age: 58
Starting weight: 275 lbs.
Current weight: 184 lbs.
Other: A grandma who
  finally has a lap for the
  grandkids to sit on!

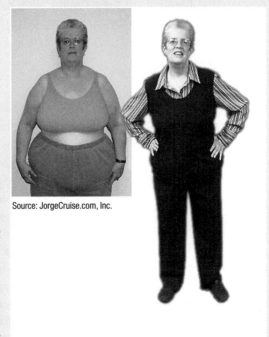

Source: JorgeCruise.com, Inc.

"Before I started the 3-Hour Diet™, I rarely looked in the mirror. I took glimpses of myself to check that the clothes were in the right place, but that was about it.

"On the 3-Hour Diet™, I established a set routine. During my work week, I roll out of bed by 5:45 a.m. so I can get in my exercises first thing. Breakfast is 6:30, and I'm on my way to work by 7:30. Snack is 10 a.m., lunch is at 1 p.m., a treat at 4, and dinner by 7. I take my book to bed around 10, and read a bit before sleep.

"I'm rather fond of dinner. **I've discovered the art of oven-roasting vegetables, and vegetables that were just okay before are now wonderful.** I do this for most evening meals. I have my portion of fresh vegetables (green beans, cauliflower, asparagus, or broccoli—sometimes with onion slices on top) that I put on a cookie sheet, slice up a couple of small red-skin potatoes, and sprinkle it all with extra virgin olive oil. I throw on Mrs. Dash®—maybe some dill—and put in the oven at 450 degrees for 20 minutes. I add some protein, and I'm set.

"This schedule has helped me to lose quite a bit of weight. It's amazing. I now actually primp in front of the mirror. I'm now buying plus sizes at regular clothing stores instead of super sizes. I'm proud of myself."

Deborah's Secrets to Success

➤ Get up early to face the day, even on the weekends.
➤ Make sure there's plenty of the right foods in your fridge and cabinets.

> Portion out your snacks into zip-lock bags so you can grab them when you're on the run.
> Always keep a meal in the freezer, just in case you get home late and need to make something fast.

Create Your Support Pillars

For every challenge in life, we all need support. It's hard to go it alone, and weight loss is no different. To be successful on this program, you must do a little homework. It will help you to start the program with the highest probability of success.

First, you are going to create what I call *support pillars*. These pillars act just like the support pillars for a building. They will prop you up and help you stand secure during any challenge. Too many people take on a weight-loss challenge without creating these pillars. Instead, they sabotage themselves by thinking negative thoughts. They remember all of the times they screwed up and all of the diets that didn't work, whether it was cabbage soup, low-carb, or something else. They tell themselves they'll try this new diet, but if it doesn't work out, it's no big deal.

That's no way to commit to a program! You must focus on your successes, not on your failures. Only when you focus on your past successes will you find the motivation to stand firm during any weight-loss challenge.

To do so, I want you to do the following:

Step 1: Think back over your life. When have you been successful? What challenges did you face that you thought you would never surmount, but eventually did? Perhaps you never thought you would get your driver's license, or move out of your parents' home into your own apartment. Maybe you thought you could never finish high school or college. Perhaps you thought you would never meet the man or woman of your dreams.

Do a brain dump. Think back over your life and write down every successful challenge in the space provided on the next page where it says "my support pillars." Then, once you are done, move on to step 2.

Step 2: Take a close look at all of your positive accomplishments. I want you to go through your list and pick your top three. Then, beside each one, write how you did it. For example, to earn your high school or college diploma, you had to show up for classes, do your homework, and study for

My Support Pillars

Write down all the positive accomplishments you can think of on the lines below:

_____

_____

_____

_____

Write your top three accomplishments (your support pillars) here along with how you accomplished each:

_____

_____

_____

1. My Pillar: _____

How I accomplished it: _____

_____

_____

_____

_____

2. My Pillar: _____

How I accomplished it: _____

_____

_____

_____

_____

3. My Pillar: _____

How I accomplished it: _____

_____

_____

_____

_____

tests. This all took a commitment, patience, and perseverance on your part. It's this same type of commitment that you need to successfully lose weight. Remember: if you think you can, you will. Focus on your past successes and you'll create a better future.

Create Your New "Name Tag"

Whatever you call yourself is how you feel about yourself. If you think of yourself as "fatso," you'll unconsciously do things—like overeat—to make yourself fat. If you think of yourself as a "hot mama," you'll do things to create that image. It's that simple.

I want you to pick a "name tag"—something to call yourself—that's positive and encourages you to meet your goal. Your new name tag will help you achieve your goal because it will motivate you about eating well. Too many people unconsciously label themselves in ways that make them feel bad. They describe themselves as old farts, over-the-hill, chubby, overeaters, emotional eaters, couch potatoes, sugar-a-holics, and so on. The human brain is such a powerful instrument that you will eventually become whatever you label yourself. For example, if you really think that you have a sweet tooth, you will always have problems with sweets. The truth is that nobody really has a sweet tooth—not any more than anyone else. It is just a saying that becomes real only when you take it on, when you own it.

Select a positive name tag for yourself. Make up something that works for you. Perhaps it's sexy mama or Adonis or hot babe or power woman. Choose something that fits, that you like, and that resonates with you deep inside. Then take on this label and make it real for you. You might ask your partner to refer to you by your new name tag, or you might write it on a piece of paper and secure it to your refrigerator. Do whatever you need to do to feel that this is your new name—and the new you.

Once you do, then you're ready to move on to chapter 5 and discover all the details of when to eat—and lose weight once and for all. Are you ready? Let's move on to the first big secret of getting thin!

SECRET 1—THE 3-HOUR TIMELINE™

Before I met Jorge Cruise, I was on a journey heading for the grave. I weighed 340 pounds and my cardio blood profile was horrible. My doctor told me I had no choice but to lose the weight. The 3-Hour Diet™ helped me control my eating. The fear of dying was and is with me, so I have no temptation to stray off the program. Anytime that I am tempted, I just remember why I am doing this program. I always remember that I am doing this for me first. After working this plan for thirty-three weeks I have lost 67 pounds. My doctor saw the results and told me that this was the best he has seen in me in over fifteen years. His exact comment was, 'Whatever you are doing, keep it up.' "Thanks to Jorge Cruise, I have my life back and I am never going back to where I once was. Thanks, Jorge."

—DON THOMPSON—LOST 67 POUNDS

When my son, Parker, was born, it changed my life—for the better. It also changed my way to think about the world. Suddenly my wife, Heather, and I found ourselves thrust into this tiny baby's powerful rhythms and away from the rhythm of life as we had known it. My wife found herself attending to Parker's needs throughout the day and night. You could almost match his hunger cries to the clock.

Although we soon both felt more fatigued than we had in a very long time, we knew this feeding schedule was important to Parker's growth and health.

This experience with Parker reminded me that there is a rhythm and schedule to everything in life. We all perform better during the day if we go to bed and get up at a set time every day. We make appointments for set days and times—and expect the people we are meeting to be on time. Most of us feel calmer and more secure if our days follow a routine: we get out of bed, brush our teeth, eat breakfast, head to work, and so on. Keeping this predictable routine is what keeps us sane.

Nature is no different. Morning glories open when the sun rises and close when it sets. In some climates, the leaves change colors every fall. Birds migrate along the same paths at the same time of year, every year. And many animals, from deer to wolves to bears, travel the same paths at the same times every day as they search for food.

Indeed, schedules are very important. The time of day that we tackle certain tasks is also important. Scientists now know, for example, that certain medications are more effective at certain times a day. They've discovered that exercising in the morning delivers more results than doing it in the afternoon or evening. And they know that many people can learn and remember information better at certain times of the day.

How does this relate to losing weight? Well, the bottom line is this: **When you eat is critical.** It's as critical as what you eat. When you eat at the right times, you will see 2 pounds of fat disappear every week and you'll keep that weight off long term. When you eat at the wrong times, you slow your metabolism, and gain weight over the long term.

Eating every 3 hours is very important. In this chapter, I hope to convince you of that fact. I will also show you that doing so need not be laborious. My 3-Hour Timeline™ technique will make timing your meals effortless.

Point 1: The 3-hour reasons

The first thing most of my online clients ask me is, "Jorge, why eat every 3 hours and not every 5 hours or every 2?" I tell them that 3 hours is the magic number that works. Thousands of my clients and many university studies back up the power of 3 hours. Then clients ask, "What will I specifically gain from spacing out my calories so that I am eating intentionally and not accidentally?" **I tell everyone that they will see up to 2 pounds disappear each week, and that they'll lose their belly fat first.** They are always amazed that this will happen. Finally, they ask me, "How does this work?" I am now going to share with you all the reasons why you will lose 2 pounds a week, and the various research studies that back this up.

Turns off the starvation protection mechanism

The number one reason I ask my clients to eat every 3 hours is to get them to force their body to turn off their starvation protection mechanism (SPM). As I already mentioned, when your SPM is off you preserve lean muscle tissue and thus preserve your resting metabolism.

Here's how the SPM works: Anytime you let more then 3 hours pass between eating episodes, you turn on the SPM. Once this happens, your body conserves fat and burns muscle. The SPM is designed to preserve the most calorie-rich tissue on the human body—body fat—to help you survive a famine. Yep, you see, thousands of years ago our bodies had to adapt to a "feast or famine" existence. When rain was plentiful and hunting was good, our ancient ancestors feasted on meat, berries, nuts, and other foods. At other times, when rain was scarce, they went days or weeks without food. To survive, the body developed a way to conserve fat during famine. When it sensed food was scarce, the body developed the ability to turn down the metabolism and conserve fat. This ensured survival by holding on to body fat as an insurance policy.

To make up for the calories lost from fat, the body taps into its own muscles as a source of energy. Why? When you go a long time without eating, your body will still need calories to function properly. This causes your muscles to cannibalize themselves, breaking down in order to provide your body the energy it needs since there is a lack of food. End result: your body cannibalizes your muscle tissue, and your metabolism plummets.

One of my favorite studies was done at Georgia State University with Olympic athletes. It found that when the athletes timed their meals and snacks with precision, it not only made them stronger and faster, but it also made them leaner. Proper timing helped increase their energy levels, alertness, and muscle mass. And here's the best news: you don't have to be an

Olympic athlete to benefit from meal timing. The tactic works for regular everyday folks, too.

There's a popular nutritional axiom that goes like this: If the calories you eat equal the calories you burn, your weight will remain stable. If the calories you eat total more than the calories you burn, you'll gain weight. Finally, if the calories you eat are less than what you burn, you'll lose weight. The axiom makes sense most of the time, but it isn't as black and white as it sounds. In the study conducted at Georgia State, female runners and gymnasts who didn't eat for more than 3 hours at a time had the highest body fat percentages (the percentage of body fat to lean tissue), even if they weren't consuming more calories than they were burning. The longer an athlete went between meals, the higher the body fat percentage.

Here are additional studies that support the beneficial effects of good meal timing.

- In a study published in the *British Journal of Nutrition*, weight loss participants who ate frequent meals preserved considerably more lean muscle tissue than participants who ate fewer daily meals but consumed the same number of calories.
- Scandinavian researchers arrived at similar results when they tested two diets on a group of athletes who were trying to lose weight. Although all of them lost the same amount of weight, the ones who ate fewer meals lost mostly lean muscle tissue, whereas the ones who ate more frequent meals lost almost all fat tissue.
- Similarly, at Nagoya University in Japan, athletes who ate frequently—six meals a day—preserved their muscle tissue as they lost weight, whereas the ones who ate the same number of calories in just two daily meals lost muscle tissue.
- And one of my favorite clinical trials was reported in the *Journal of Human Clinical Nutrition*: weight loss increased and the loss of lean muscle was minimized in a group of obese woman who ate every 3 hours, versus another group of obese women who ate every 6 hours!

This is why eating *every 3 hours* is so important. It helps to keep that starvation protection system turned off, and your metabolism turned on. Hopefully you are thinking, "Sounds good to me, Jorge . . . I am convinced." Well, I am not going to stop. You see, there are even MORE extraordinary benefits to eating every 3 hours.

Increases basal metabolic rate

When you spread your calories out over the course of the day, you feed your body energy as it needs it. This allows your cells to quickly take up blood sugar as it becomes available, and burn it for energy. When you eat fewer meals—and more calories at those meals—your body cannot use as many calories as you consume. So it stores the excess in your fat cells.

End result: You gain weight, even though you may be eating the same number of calories during the course of the day.

Eating frequent meals helps you burn calories in other ways as well. Your body burns calories after every meal as it churns food up in your stomach and pushes it through your intestines. Researchers call this post-meal calorie burn the *thermic effect of food*. In a study completed at Queens Medical Center in the United Kingdom, study participants who ate six meals a day had a higher thermic effect of food than participants who ate fewer meals per day. In another study completed at the University of Nottingham, also in the UK, participants who ate sporadically and erratically burned fewer calories as they digested their food compared to participants who ate frequently and regularly. Although the number of extra calories burned is not high, it can certainly help you shed the fat!

Increases energy levels

Have you ever felt really tired during the late afternoon? This is often a result of going too long without food. When you go too long without food, blood sugar levels drop and you hit the wall. You can't think clearly and you want to take a nap.

When you eat every 3 hours, however, you keep blood sugar levels stable and provide a steady flow of amino acids and sugar to feed muscle and brain tissue. This steadies your moods and boosts your energy. You'll have a steady supply of energy all day long.

Besides making you feel better, this increased energy can further fuel your weight loss because you will become more active automatically. Think about it. When you are tired, you find ways to move less. You take the elevator instead of the stairs. You send an e-mail rather than walking to a coworker's office. You take a nap rather than taking a walk. When you have more energy, however, you'll find yourself taking walking breaks at work—because they feel good!

Suppresses appetite—naturally

When I first tell my clients about the wonders of meal timing, some of them worry that they will eat more—and eat too much—if they eat every 3 hours. This couldn't be further from the truth.

When you feed your body every 3 hours, you keep blood sugar levels stable, which automatically suppresses your appetite. In the studies conducted at Georgia State, mentioned earlier, athletes automatically ate less at every meal once they switched to the every-three-hour way of eating. All of my clients feel the same way. Other research shows that people who eat more frequent meals have fewer cravings and binge less often because they don't feel as hungry when it's time to eat. Again, all my clients and I agree.

In a wonderful study completed in the Netherlands, obese women who ate more frequent meals had more optimal levels of leptin hormones. What is leptin? It is a hormone produced by fat cells that plays a major role in suppressing appetite. Bottom line: these women felt less hungry and had fewer cravings throughout the day. Also, researchers in Johannesburg, South Africa fed obese men either five meals over the course of the day or one huge meal. Men who ate only once a day consumed 27 percent more calories than those who ate more frequently.

Think of the last time you felt really, really hungry and then went out to eat at a restaurant. Were your eyes bigger than your stomach? Did you order more food than usual, eat faster than usual, and eat so much food that you felt swollen and sick later? I bet you did. Most people do.

Many of my clients who had struggled with emotional eating before they came to me have found that such hurdles became much smaller once they tried the 3-Hour Diet™. "We have been going through a very stressful time in our household—personal family issues, remodeling our home, and making major investments," Victoria Brown, told me. "Normally I would be comfort-fooding myself through this. Instead I'm able to focus on the stressful issues and not let it get out of control, knowing my next meal or snack is just 3 hours away or less. I'm not focused on food, rather I'm planning for it. I'm not starving myself or punishing myself."

Another one of my clients, Teresa Neal, says eating every 3 hours helps her to stick to a healthier diet. "I don't eat outside of the 3-Hour Diet™ plan because I always know I'm going to be eating again in just 3 hours," she told me. "I never have trouble ordering in restaurants anymore. I always can hold out for 3 hours. I'm happy with the results I'm seeing, and that truly is motivational."

Another client, Karen Taporco, says eating regularly has helped her to avoid unplanned snacking—and hundreds of excess calories. "Eating every 3 hours helps me avoid unplanned snacking. It's allowed me to develop a routine so that choosing the right food becomes second nature."

Lowers cholesterol

Yes, eating every 3 hours helps keep your cholesterol levels low, too. It turns out your cholesterol level depends not only on what you eat, but also on how often you eat. In a study just reported in the *British Medical Journal*, it was shown that people who eat six or more times a day have cholesterol levels that are about 5 percent lower than those of less-frequent eaters. And this was true regardless of body mass, physical activity, or whether they smoked or not. According to the study, when you eat larger meals and go for longer periods of time between meals, insulin peaks at higher levels. High peaks of insulin alter fat and cholesterol metabolism, producing higher levels of cholesterol in your blood. Frequent small meals control insulin secretion and prevent these peaks. The result: lower levels of cholesterol. I should point out that a 5 percent reduction in cholesterol levels doesn't sound like much, but it does have a large impact on your risk for heart disease since it reduces coronary artery disease by 10 percent!

Reduces the belly-bulging hormone cortisol

The New England Journal of Medicine published a wonderful study by the Department of Nutritional Sciences in Toronto, Canada, that specifically showed how eating every 3 hours helped reduce levels of the stress hormone cortisol. You see, high cortisol hormone levels are closely associated to abdominal fat. In the study it was shown that in as little as two weeks, individuals who ate frequent, small meals as opposed to three large meals (containing the same total amount of food) were able to reduce their cortisol levels by more than 17 percent. Truly amazing, isn't it? And all these benefits occurred in only two weeks! Just imagine what a lifetime of eating this way will do for you.

Point 2: The 3-hour daily rules

There are three daily rules that I tell my clients are the foundational keys to success with the 3-Hour Diet™.

1. Reconnect to the science
2. Develop a mental timeline (the night before or at breakfast)
3. Commit your timeline to paper

The first key to your success will be to reconnect each day with the scientific benefits you just learned in the previous section. Yep, too often we forget *why* we do something and thus we stop. It is very important to know and remember that by eating every 3 hours you are preserving your lean muscle and metabolism, that you are increasing your basal metabolic rate, that you are boosting your energy, that you are suppressing your appetite, lowering your cholesterol, and even reducing your cortisol levels. To help you remember all this, photocopy the reminder sheet [on the next page] and post it on your refrigerator, your office cubicle, and/or at your bedside. Put it in as many places as you can. Each morning reconnect to this list before you start your day to keep you motivated and eating!

The second key is to develop a mental timeline in your head of when you are going to eat. That means thinking, "Well, if I am eating breakfast at 7 a.m.; that means that 10 a.m. is my snack, then lunch is at 1 p.m., then my second snack is at 4 p.m., with dinner at 7 p.m., followed shortly thereafter with a treat." I usually recommend you do this either just before you go to bed or first thing in the morning when you are eating breakfast.

The last key is to finally commit your mental timeline to paper. This is critical, or you will forget and lose track of your eating. To do this you will use chapter 9 where you will have four weeks of my 3-Hour Timeline™ system to keep you organized and on track. What exactly is my Cruise Timeline™? Well, it is my secret weapon to help you eat effortlessly all throughout the day.

Point 3: The 3-Hour Timeline™

I want to share with you a simple visual technique that I've developed that will help you seamlessly incorporate the 3-Hour Diet™ into your lifestyle.

When I first designed the 3-Hour Diet™ and tested it on my online clients, I got a lot of feedback. They all loved the diet and achieved great success. But some of them told me that they had trouble remembering when to eat. They would get caught up in meetings at work, or rush from one errand to another. At the end of the day they'd realize that they missed a snack or even an entire meal.

Because of this, I spent of a lot of time thinking about how could I help

Your 3-Hour Reasons Reminder Sheet

NOTE: Photocopy this reminder sheet and review each morning to stay motivated and eating!

1. Turns off your starvation protection mechanism (SPM), which preserves lean muscle . . . and thus preserves your resting metabolism.
2. Increases basal metabolic rate
3. Increases energy levels
4. Suppresses appetite
5. Lowers cholesterol
6. Reduces the belly-bulging hormone cortisol

my clients make eating every 3 hours automatic. I stumbled upon some studies about how humans are *visual* creatures. It just made sense. When something is in sight, it's in your mind. When it's out of sight, it's out of your mind. That's why many of us like to display the papers we need on top of our desk rather than file them away. It's also why many people leave vitamins out on a counter rather than putting them away in a cabinet. When they see those papers, they remember to fill them out. When they see their vitamins, they remember to take them.

I also talked with my most successful clients and found that they were already using some sort of *visual* system to make eating automatic. Many of them were logging their mealtimes during the day with a journal or diary. I wanted to take what I learned from them, the studies I had read, and what I knew from experience to design a visual logging system that all of my clients—and now you—could use to make timing easier. I call this visual system the 3-Hour Timeline™.

Many, many others have capitalized on the power of visual images. Newspapers like *USA Today* use many graphics and other visual images to convey information in a way that more people can understand. Most of us prefer to get information from television or the Internet—because they are visual—rather than from a book or an audio tape (Unless, of course, that book has some great drawings, picture or images—like this one).

Because humans are such visual beings, it seemed only natural to create a visual system to help my clients remember when and what to eat. I knew

KAREN TAPORCO—LOST 36 POUNDS (AND 20 INCHES)

Height: 5'3"
Age: 34
Starting weight: 175 lbs.
Current weight: 139 lbs.
Other: Married full-time
professional

Before I started Jorge's 3-Hour Diet™, I had tried and failed at weight loss many times. It seemed as if I was always dieting, but never making any real progress. I felt frumpy. I would hide behind huge, baggy clothes and hated to shop because nothing ever fit my disproportioned shape. I would not be caught wearing a pair of shorts, so I suffered through a hot summer just to hide my chunky legs. I fell into

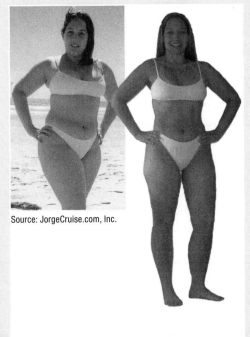

Source: JorgeCruise.com, Inc.

a sedentary lifestyle where food became my pastime pleasure.

"It wasn't until the Jorge Cruise plan that I learned to eat balanced meals. Nothing was off-limits, although I had to be mindful of how much to eat and when to eat it. **Finally, I could control my once out-of-control appetite by eating every 3 hours.** I have learned to incorporate this method into my daily life. I now know what it takes and how to make it happen.

"I had never realized how many calories were in some of the fast food and junk food choices I would make on a weekly basis. There were many times I would eat as many calories in one meal as I am now eating in an entire day. I am amazed that I do not crave those bad foods any more, and that I am comfortable knowing how to make the right choices. This has definitely been an easy program to follow and I have seen amazing results. Who knew it could be this easy and enjoyable?"

Karen's Secrets to Success

> ➤ Plan breakfast time based on a certain event for the day. For example, if, I have a business luncheon at noon, I eat breakfast at 6 a.m., followed by my snack 3 hours later.
> ➤ Keep a freezer full of frozen entrees, so you can grab a quick meal without much preparation.

I needed a visual picture, but I still wasn't quite sure what it should look like.

And then it struck me. I remembered a few months back when I visited the CNN headquarters in Atlanta. As I walked in, I couldn't help but notice a huge *timeline* that detailed many of the historical events that had been reported by CNN. The timeline pictures everything from CNN's launch in 1980 to major events the news channel had covered, such as the Columbia space shuttle disaster and Ronald Reagan's shooting. It was so visual that it was easy to see and remember the important events that had taken place over time. Thinking back to that day, I was amazed at how much of the timeline I could remember. As I mentioned earlier, I have a bad memory. It impressed me that simply seeing images on a timeline could improve my ability to recall information so powerfully.

And that's when it hit me. What worked for CNN could work for the 3-Hour Diet™. So I went to work, designing a timeline that my clients could use to remember when to eat. I tested it over and over on various clients and went through many different versions. I finally created one that everyone loved. More important, it really helped them see when to eat and, thus, helped them eat on time! Mission accomplished. I found that my clients who used the timeline religiously never forgot their schedule. They always ate on time!

That's why I'm so convinced that the 3-Hour Timeline™ will help you make eating on time automatic and effortless. In addition to creating a visual image, the process of writing down what you will eat—and when you will eat it—will help to reinforce your commitment to eating every 3 hours.

And, don't worry. You won't have to do this forever. By the end of the first twenty-eight days, the 3-Hour Diet™ will have become automatic for you. You will have trained your body—and your brain—to eat every 3 hours. You will no longer have trouble remembering to fit in a meal. Your stomach will tell you: "I'm hungry. Feed me." You'll have formed an important habit that will help you lose weight and keep it off!

How to use the timeline

This timeline will help you see at a glance what you will be eating each day and when you will be eating it. This visual image will help reinforce the concept of Visual Timing™, putting a visual picture in your mind that will help you to stay on track (see next page for a sample). For the first twenty-eight days of the program in chapter 9, you will fill in that day's timeline ahead of time. I recommend you fill in your timeline the night before you start each day, or at breakfast each morning for the rest of the day. You simply write in what time you are going to eat your meals—and what you will eat (or ate). You will find three places for breakfast, lunch, and dinner, one place for your snacks, and one place for your treat at the end of the day. Also, make sure to check off your glasses of water.

You can create your own meals using the guidance of the 3-Hour Plate™ in chapter 6, or chose from my sample premade meals in chapter 13. Either way, you will write them down. Based on what time you get up in the morning, you will write in the time for each meal. You'll pick the times you eat based on the following:

1. Eat breakfast within one hour of rising.
2. Eat every 3 hours.
3. Stop eating 3 hours before bedtime.

Here's why. Let me start with breakfast. To keep your metabolism running strong, you must eat your first meal within one hour of rising. As you sleep, your body is not getting any food, and consequently turns down your metabolism. When you awake, you want to kick your metabolism back into high gear as soon as possible. If you don't eat within one hour of waking, your body will protect the most precious calorie-rich tissue in your body that it will need to survive during a famine—body fat. It turns down your metabolism even more and begins to cannibalize muscle instead of fat tissue. So if you skip breakfast, you just end up hurting up your efforts.

This, as you've seen, is the same reasoning behind why you should eat every 3 hours. Frequent meals will help keep your metabolism running smoothly for the rest of the day. The key is eating five times throughout the day, separated by 3 hours. In other words, this means you might eat breakfast at 7 a.m., have a snack at 10 a.m., eat lunch at 1 p.m., then have another snack at 4 p.m., and finally eat dinner at 7 p.m. with a treat

Your 3-Hour Plan

1) Commit your eating times.
2) Create your custom meals from the food lists starting on page 268 or from the premade meals starting on page 283.
3) Then keep your eye on this page and check off boxes when done eating.

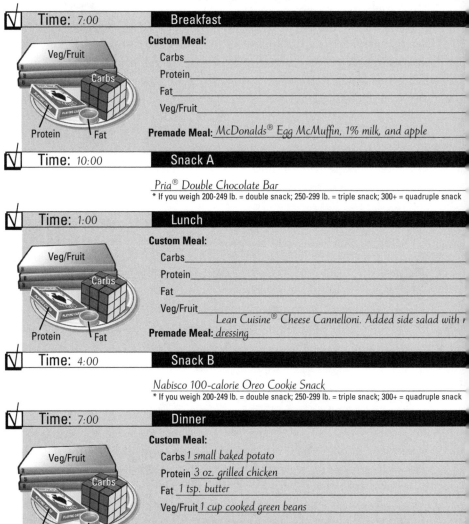

☑ **Time:** 7:00 — **Breakfast**

Custom Meal:
Carbs_____
Protein_____
Fat_____
Veg/Fruit_____

Premade Meal: *McDonalds® Egg McMuffin, 1% milk, and apple*

☑ **Time:** 10:00 — **Snack A**

Pria® Double Chocolate Bar
* If you weigh 200-249 lb. = double snack; 250-299 lb. = triple snack; 300+ = quadruple snack

☑ **Time:** 1:00 — **Lunch**

Custom Meal:
Carbs_____
Protein_____
Fat_____
Veg/Fruit_____

Premade Meal: *Lean Cuisine® Cheese Cannelloni. Added side salad with dressing*

☑ **Time:** 4:00 — **Snack B**

Nabisco 100-calorie Oreo Cookie Snack
* If you weigh 200-249 lb. = double snack; 250-299 lb. = triple snack; 300+ = quadruple snack

☑ **Time:** 7:00 — **Dinner**

Custom Meal:
Carbs *1 small baked potato*
Protein *3 oz. grilled chicken*
Fat *1 tsp. butter*
Veg/Fruit *1 cup cooked green beans*

Premade Meal:_____

☑ **Time:** 10:00 — **Treat**

12 M&M's

Water

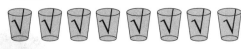

Freebie Tracker
1 Diet Coke
1 cup coffee
1 nondairy liquid creamer

shortly thereafter or 3 hours later (that's up to you). This is a perfect eating schedule, and I strongly recommend you follow this time pattern closely.

What if you get out of bed later or earlier than 7 a.m.? Then pick your meal times based on the time you rise. If you get out of bed at 9 a.m., then eat breakfast by 10 a.m. and follow the schedule to eat every three hours from there. Don't worry if you miss a meal by 10 or 15 minutes. A metabolism alarm isn't going to sound off exactly when 3 hours have passed. However, you do want to stick to this schedule as *closely* as you can for the best results.

Finally, let's talk about why you should stop eating 3 hours before bedtime. When the sun goes down each day, your body's temperature begins to drop, and vital functions like heartbeat and breathing begin to slow down, readying you for sleep. If you can eat in a way that supports this natural rhythm, you will ensure that your body gets a full night's rest. If you eat just before bedtime, you take too much food to bed with you, your digestive system keeps you awake as it breaks down your food and your body spends its energy on digestion rather than on repairing and firming your lean muscle tissues. Though you may actually be able to fall asleep, you won't sleep as deeply while your body digests food. And you need deep sleep in order for your body to truly rest and recover. Your goal is to make sure that you recuperate during sleep rather than waste your rest on digestion. I promise you will feel more energized and alive when you wake!

More tips to make it happen

My 3-Hour Timeline™ will help to ensure that you stick with the 3-Hour Diet™. But you can do even more to ensure your success. In addition to consistently filling in and looking at your visual timeline each day, I want you to choose one more technique that will help you remember to eat every 3 hours. Consider it a gentle tap on the shoulder—reminding you that you must eat to keep your metabolism running strong.

The following techniques have worked for many of my clients:

Get a watch with a countdown timer. Many of my clients set their watches to beep every 3 hours. When their alarm goes off, it reminds them of their #1 priority: eating every 3 hours. Whether they are in a meeting, changing a baby's diaper, or doing something else, they know they must soon stop what they are doing and eat a meal or a snack.

Put it in your electronic calendar. Many of my clients use a cell phone, PDA, or their personal computer to write down their daily schedule. These devices then beep to remind them of each daily appointment. In addition to inserting their dentist appointments, important meetings, and upcoming birthdays into these electronic calendars, they also type in their meal schedule. That way, the calendar will remind them when to eat. This method also helps many of my clients to see ahead of time if another appointment will conflict with their eating schedule and to plan accordingly. For example, when one of my clients realized she was going to be stuck in a four-hour meeting at work, she brought a yogurt smoothie from our snack list to the meeting—expertly hidden in a coffee cup! Everyone at the meeting thought she was sipping coffee, but she was really having one of her snacks!

Find an accountability buddy. Telling a trusted friend about your goal to eat every 3 hours will help to keep you honest. You might pick a family member or a co-worker. Or, you can go online to www.JorgeCruise.com and find a buddy on my website. This person will ask you how the diet is going each day. Just the thought that you will have to check in will help fuel your motivation to stay on track. The pressure will be to eat on time because your buddy may be checking up on you!

Use the JorgeCruise.com planner. If you join our online club, you will get full access to our online eating planners. Each week you can print a personalized visual eating packet to keep you superorganized, and much more.

SIX

SECRET 2—THE 3-HOUR PLATE™

live in a beautiful condominium, with antiques and beautifully carved mother of pearl screens, and yet I've made sure the mirrors in my unit are in locations where I don't have to look at myself. Until I met Jorge, I was on a yearly downward spiral, gaining pounds each year. I felt grossly lethargic. I never realized how important and how essential it is to eat. I am down 11 pounds in just five weeks on Jorge's 3-Hour Diet™. I feel my metabolism kicking in, I feel my stomach digesting, I have energy and I like how I feel. I've now gone out and bought a full-length mirror."

—DENA DEAN—LOST 11 POUNDS

I have wonderful news: you will actually lose weight *more easily* by breaking out of the forbidden-food trap and eating the very foods you crave. Ready to get really smart? If you've been turning the other cheek to cheesecake, blowing off pasta, or missing out on Jack in the Box®, it's time to stop depriving yourself, because deprivation always leads to weight gain in the long run.

This means on the 3-Hour Diet™ you will never have to ban foods or deprive yourself of any food—ever. Why? If you deprive yourself of the things you like, then eventually you will binge and you'll sabotage your success. This is the second secret to Visual Timing™. Yep, I tell my online clients the secret to being successful long term is you must make your meals *tempting*. YES!! That's why you now must discover how to easily eat without restricting food options—ever. By doing this you will ensure you consistently lose 2 pounds every week. Plus, you will be able to keep the weight off long-term, and most importantly, truly bring back the joy of eating into your life.

So get ready because with the 3-Hour Diet™

You will be able to eat anywhere. My online client Mary used to eat at her desk every day. Her coworkers would ask her to join them for lunch in the cafeteria or at a local restaurant, but she knew she couldn't survive the temptation, and she didn't want people she worked with to see her eat too much. But with the 3-Hour Diet™, Mary was prepared with a prepacked lunch, and she was armed with knowledge about good choices and self-control when the group ate out. With the 3-Hour Diet™, never again will you have to substitute salad for Thanksgiving dinner, and your mother's extra-chocolatey cake will no longer be a no-no on your birthday. And the buffet table at the neighborhood picnic? Bring it on. You now will have the smarts to dish up the right portions of what you love and enjoy—without sabotaging yourself.

You will have total freedom. When there are no banned foods in your life, you won't have to devote so much energy to thinking about what you can't have. Because you possess the necessary skills, you will be empowered to tackle any eating situation with poise. Like Mary, you will never have to avoid a social eating situation again. You'll be the person people look at and say, "Where does she put it?"

So say goodbye to deprivation. The 3-Hour Diet™ will tempt your taste buds by including your favorite foods, drawing you to eat healthful portions automatically. You will look forward to eating like never before and thus, will be able to make the 3-Hour Diet™ a *lifestyle*.

In this chapter you will learn how to eat with my 3-Hour Plate™ which

The 3-Hour Solution

By eating balanced portions of proteins, fats, and carbohydrates, you will:

- Release yourself from the guilt of deprivation dieting
- Reduce cravings and binges
- Feel in control of your eating
- Be able to eat any food—anywhere—and stick to your diet

visually teaches you how to eat the right amounts of the foods you love, without counting calories or adding up points or grams. In chapter 12 and 13 you'll find food lists and meal ideas that make it even easier for you to select many different kinds of quick and easy meals, snacks, and treats. They include homemade meals, frozen foods, and even meals from Jack in the Box® and McDonalds® to Taco Bell® and KFC® fast-food restaurants. That's right. Even fast food is not off-limits on the 3-Hour Diet™.

Get ready to bring back the joy of eating!

What you will eat

The goal is to follow a healthy eating plan that helps you eat the foods you really enjoy in the right amounts, in a way that supports muscle growth and boosts your metabolism. On this plan you will eat three meals, two snacks, and one delicious treat *every day.* During those meals, you will eat a variety of foods that fall into the big three food categories called *macronutrients*: carbohydrates, fats and proteins. Carbohydrates and fats supply your body's caloric needs, and proteins repair body tissues. In addition, you need vitamins and minerals, in the form of fruits, vegetables and dietary supplements, to fight disease and boost your metabolism. Each meal on the 3-Hour Diet™ balances these nutrients for maximum health and weight loss.

Each of the following three food groups is a crucial part of your success.

Food Group 1: Carbohydrates

Carbohydrates come from plants that house sugar, starch, or fiber. This includes sugar cane (which is turned into table sugar and various sweeteners), grains (such as wheat), and fruits and vegetables. Your body converts these sugars and starches into blood sugar (called glucose) and transports it to cells to be burned for energy. The most efficient energy source for the body, carbohydrates supply between 40 and 50 percent of the body's energy needs when you are at rest (not exercising). Unlike fats and proteins, the body can break these nutrients down almost instantly and use them for energy.

And that brings me to the first all-important reason why you need to eat carbs: Carbohydrates are important because they provide the fuel necessary to keep your lean muscles healthy. When you skimp on carbs your muscles shrivel up, your energy plummets, and you move less and less. All this makes you cannibalize your lean muscle tissues, causing you to burn fewer calories. Make sure to review chapter 2 for more details about the impact of low carbohydrates in your body.

Carbohydrates are also critical for healthy digestion. Many carbohydrate foods contain fiber, pectin, and other nutrients that help slow digestion, allowing you to feel fuller on less food. They also help keep things moving in your intestines, which not only prevents constipation but also reduces the calories absorbed by your intestines into your bloodstream.

On the 3-Hour Diet™, you can eat any carbohydrate. It's true. You can have cake, crackers, bagels, or pasta. But you should know that some carbohydrates will help fuel your weight loss even further. These are "whole" carbs.

Carbohydrates fall into two main categories: whole and refined. Whole carbohydrates are the best. They're grains in their whole form, which means they still contain their outer shell, and they haven't been bleached or overly processed.

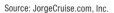

This outer shell contains fiber that helps slow digestion, helping you feel full on less food. The more slowly a food digests, the more slowly it turns into sugar in your bloodstream, and the more it acts as a fuel to burn body fat. When you eat whole carbohydrates, your body gets a steady, time-released sugar, so you never get

Source: JorgeCruise.com, Inc.

Why You Must Eat Carbs

Carbohydrates are crucial to your weight-loss success. You need carbs to

1. Maintain muscle growth, so your metabolism will remain strong
2. Boost your energy levels, so you'll move more often and burn more calories as a result
3. Improve digestion, so you'll stay regular

overwhelmed with sugar rushes and your body will use fat as its primary fuel!

Whole carbohydrates include whole grains like oats and brown rice, oatmeal, 100 percent whole-grain bread, and high-fiber whole grain breakfast cereals. You don't *have to* eat these foods on the 3-Hour Diet™. Consider it extra credit. If you do stick to whole carbs most of the time, you'll fuel your weight loss even more.

Although you can eat them on the 3-Hour Diet™, refined carbohydrates are not quite as good as the whole variety. They include white rice and bread, instant hot cereals, and some low-fiber, high-sugar cold cereals. To make them easier to cook and not so bland, the food industry strips carbohydrates of their natural fiber content, pulverizing them into smaller pieces. Because they are refined, your body digests these carbohydrates more quickly than it does whole carbohydrates.

To visualize the difference between whole and refined carbohydrates, think of a campfire where the logs represent your body fat. To get maximum heat, you would light the big logs by using kindling and a little bit of lighter fluid, causing the logs to burn slowly and steadily for a long time. Whole carbohydrates are like the kindling and refined carbohydrates are like lighter fluid.

If you only eat refined carbohydrates, it would be like only pouring lighter fluid onto the logs, causing a fast fire that burns out almost immediately. Your ideal goal would be to include whole carbs as often as possible.

A good way to gauge whether a carbohydrate is whole or refined is to check the nutrition facts label. Foods that contain three or more grams of fiber per serving are more whole than those foods that contain less fiber. And remember: because there are no banned foods, you don't have to elim-

Age: 40
Starting Weight: 310 lbs.
Current Weight: 155 lbs.
Other: Happily married
  stay-at-home mom of
  three children

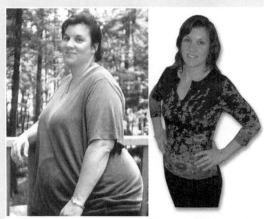

Source: JorgeCruise.com, Inc.

"The image I used to see in the mirror before I started Jorge Cruise was not me. I did not know who that person was. I felt as if I was wearing a sign for all the world to see that said 'undisciplined woman who can't lose weight.' Everyday, I was constantly thinking about my weight. I would tell myself, 'I need to do something,' 'tomorrow I will be good,' 'I'll never be able to lose over a hundred pounds' and so on. It was exhausting and draining.

"Then I discovered Jorge Cruise. From the very first day, I knew this was different. **It is amazing, how small changes over time will add up to big changes over time—155 pounds of change!** At first, I had the eating habits of a six-year-old. It was too overwhelming in the beginning to make a lot of dietary changes at once, so I made many small changes over time. First, I started drinking more water. Then, I increased my vegetable and fruit intake. I also cut down on my portion sizes.

"I also started to think about how different foods made my body feel. I realized that protein made me feel full longer. I began to notice that I felt sluggish and got a headache from too much sugar. When I ate late at night, I felt groggy in the morning. As I listened to my body, it helped me change my relationship with food. Eating every three hours also helped me to focus on what I was eating, how much I was eating, and how often I was eating. It helped me stop all the 'mindless eating' and to make better and healthier choices.

"I am now a woman who is taking charge of her health and her life. I am proud of the fact that I worked hard and sweated off every pound. When I look in the mirror now, I know the woman looking back at me!"

Maria's Secrets to Success:

➤ Make lists, plan ahead for the next day and just do it!
➤ Buy a calendar to keep track of your eating and exercise routine. Mark off every day that you exercise. Once you see all of the marks, you'll be motivated to keep it up.
➤ Add in Jorge's 8 Minute Moves® for more fat burning, toning and firming!

inate refined carbohydrates altogether. Just eat the whole ones as often as you can. For a full list of whole carbohydrates you will love, please refer to my food lists in chapter 12.

Food Group 2: Proteins

Derived from a Greek word which means "of first quality," protein is the basic material of life. It's in three-fourths of our bodily tissues; it can be found in our muscles, organs, antibodies, hormones, and enzymes. Made up of a chain of various types of amino acids—the basic building blocks of life—protein is critical to your weight loss success.

Your muscles are made of protein, so it may be no surprise to you that you must eat protein to maintain them. Without muscles you wouldn't be able to stand or burn calories, because protein is the material your body uses to create and maintain lean muscle, it's pretty important that you include protein in your daily menu. If you don't eat enough protein, your body will start to break down and recycle existing protein from your lean muscle fibers, which will cause you to lose muscle (your fat-burning machine) and slow down your metabolism. As a result, you will burn less body fat. Your muscles also form the shape of your body. So, when you eat protein you literally help to sculpt your body thin!

In addition to your muscle tissue, protein is also part of your hair, skin, and nails. By eating protein you keep your hair stronger and less likely to become damaged. Your nails will grow longer and your skin will look more radiant.

Finally, protein is critical for optimal immunity. Protein plays a key role in keeping you alive by fueling essential bodily processes such as your immune function. Protein is part of every cell in your body—and your body needs dietary protein to keep itself healthy. When you skimp on protein,

Why You Must Eat Protein

Protein fuels weight loss in the following ways:

1. Maintains your muscles, and therefore your metabolism
2. Keeps your skin, hair, and nails strong and healthy
3. Boosts your immunity, so you're sick less often and feel better overall

your body doesn't have the raw materials it needs to repair your muscles, organs, and other tissues. It would be like building a house with only half as much wood as you really need. You wouldn't have a very strong house—and it would probably blow over during the first storm. It's the same with your body. Without enough protein, your immunity plummets, and you can catch the common cold more often.

But beware, too much protein is as bad as too little! When you eat too much protein and too few carbohydrates (typical of low-carb diets), your body starts burning protein for fuel. Like leaded gasoline, protein is a dirty fuel source because it contains nitrogen. Instead of producing just water and carbon dioxide as carbohydrates do, protein produces toxic by-products, causing your body to flush out the toxic nitrogen with excess urine. Unfortunately, this urine also flushes out valuable minerals like calcium. A lot of the weight loss with high protein diets is due to water loss.

As with carbs, some types of protein will fuel your weight loss efforts more than others. For optimal weight loss, choose lean protein foods that are low in saturated (animal) fats. Good sources of lean protein include egg whites, fish, white-meat poultry, low-fat yogurt, 1 percent milk, and legumes (such as peanuts and beans). If you just have to have a high-saturated food like red meat, go ahead—remember, there are no banned foods—but choose a leaner sirloin or round cut if you can.

For a full list of recommended protein sources, please refer to my food lists in chapter 12.

Source: JorgeCruise.com, Inc.

Food Group 3: Fats

Many people fear fats because they contain the most calories per gram—9 calories per gram versus 4 for carbohydrates and proteins. While many deprivation diets shun fats, you need fats as much as you need carbohydrates and proteins! Fat is essential for many bodily processes. You must consume fat to remain healthy. Certain fats contain substances called *essential fatty acids* that cannot be manufactured inside the human body. These fatty substances, found both in animal products and some vegetables, serve as the raw materials for many hormones and muscle cell membranes. In animals, just as in humans, body fat serves as the storage location for excess calories. These fat cells can fill up and multiply, serving as a storehouse for calories and for extra insulation. You can often see these fats on various cuts of meat. Fat can also be found in dairy products, eggs, nuts and seeds, and some fruits and vegetables including avocados, olives, and coconuts.

There are many types of fat. Saturated fats are found in animal products such as steak, whole milk, and eggs. Hydrogenated fats (also called *trans fats*) are found in many processed foods. These man-made fats help extend the shelf life of many foods and were used as a replacement for saturated fats during the low-fat craze of the 1990s. I usually recommend all my clients minimize or avoid the use of these trans fats for optimal health. Finally, there are essential fatty acids, also called *omega fats*. These omega fats are true gems when it comes to weight loss.

Fats can help fuel your weight loss in three critical ways. First, and most important, omega fats help maintain healthy, lean muscle while suppressing your appetite and making you feel full on less food. Second, these omega fats help unlock stored body fat so your body can burn it for energy. Omega fats help balance your body's ratio of insulin to glucagons. Insulin signals the body to store fat, but glucagons signal the body to burn it. A diet rich in omega fats turns down insulin and turns up glucagons, so you burn fat more easily! Finally, omega fats boost your body's metabolism, so you'll burn more calories all day long. No other fat on earth will do this. Your body uses omega fats to maintain the integrity of its 75 trillion cell membranes. Having healthier cell membranes means that you improve the vehicles which transport oxygen, one of the key elements needed for fat burning. The more oxygen you have available, the easier it is for your lean muscle tissue to convert body fat into energy.

Not all fats have these important functions, however. Although you are free to eat any fats you want, you'll maximize your weight loss efforts if you

Why You Must Eat Fat

Dietary fat helps fuel weight loss by:

- Reducing your appetite
- Unlocking fat cells so more fat can be burned
- Boosting your metabolism

Source: JorgeCruise.com, Inc.

primarily try to stick with omega fats. They're also great for your overall health and youth preservation. Study after study has linked these fats with a lower risk for heart disease and certain cancers. You'll find omega fats in flaxseed products, olive oil, soybeans and other seeds, nuts (especially almonds), almond butter, olives and olive oil, fatty cold-water fish such as salmon, and avocados and guacamole.

Now, can you eat other kinds of fats? You bet. When I am at a restaurant and there is no flax oil, I will ask the server for either olive oil or butter. I like both. It's just that I try to eat flaxseed products more often, because I know they are better for my health—and my body weight.

Veggies

Your mom was right: you should eat your vegetables. Vegetables are extremely important because they're an excellent source of healthful vitamins, minerals, and phytochemicals. And they're low in calories and full of fiber so they'll fill you up without filling you out!

All vegetables contain water, but some, such as lettuce, cucumbers, sprouts, and broccoli, are particularly high in water content. The water you get from eating vegetables will increase your oxygen levels, and that oxygen will help your muscles convert fat into energy. As a result, your metabolism will be boosted.

Most raw veggies are hard and crunchy, so you have to chew them for a while. This gives your brain enough time to realize it's time to turn off

The Mighty Omegas

QUICK REFERENCE CHART

Omega-3 fats. The best type of omega fat for your health, lean muscles, and waistline, this fat is found in flax products and fatty cold-water fish such as salmon. Liquid flaxseed oil is my favorite fat of all time. I use it daily on salads or bread, and in soups (as a garnish after cooking). Since this oil is very sensitive to heat, make sure it is always fresh and refrigerated. Do not cook with this fat.

Omega-6 fats. You'll find these fats in many types of vegetable oils, such as soybean oil, safflower oil, sunflower oil, and corn oil. We consume far too many omega-6's compared to omega-3's. The omega-3's and 6's should be consumed in equal proportions. Unfortunately, we consume ten to twenty times as much omega-6 as we do omega-3. This creates an imbalance in the body that can result in inflammation, swelling, water retention, and weight gain. Try to avoid consuming excess omega-6 by limiting your ingestion of the omega-6—dominant oils listed above. Additionally, including flax oil in your daily diet will help to bring your body back to balance.

Omega-9 fats. Found in olives, avocados, and nuts, these fats are also great for your health and waistline. My second favorite fat of all time is extra virgin olive oil. I add this fat to meals when on the road because it is found almost everywhere. Olive oil is also a perfect fat for cooking.

your hunger switch. And once they're in your stomach, because of their high fiber content, vegetables are digested more slowly and make you feel full and satiated so you'll be less likely to overeat.

The reason vegetables are so low in calories is that they're low in simple sugars. You can literally eat most vegetables without restraint, and you won't put on excess pounds.

And the rich, vibrant colors of vegetables signal that they're chocked full of phytochemicals, chemicals that help keep your immune system strong and efficient. One serving of green, yellow, red, or orange vegetables may serve as many as 100 different phytochemicals—that's 100 ways for you to help prevent disease!

Source: JorgeCruise.com, Inc.

The Wonders of Flax

My all-time favorite source of fat is the omega-3 called flaxseed oil. It is the richest source of omega-3 fats (see chart on page 79) and is derived from flax seeds (also know as linseed in certain countries). Flaxseed oil is truly amazing. Your body uses it to help maintain the integrity and function of your body's 75 trillion cell membranes to support healthy joints, shiny hair and strong nails, radiant, glowing skin, and the membranes of your muscles. And because it's so widely used throughout your body, it almost never gets stored as body fat! Flaxseed oil has been shown to activate leptin, a hormone that helps suppress appetite.

My online clients consistently give me positive feedback about flaxseed oil, saying it satisfies them, makes them feel full longer, and makes their muscles feel more healthy. If that weren't enough, flaxseed oil activates a type of fat that lies deep within your body and surrounds your vital organs, called *brown fat*. Leftover from the days when we needed to brave the elements with little clothing, brown fat burns calories for heat. When you activate your brown fat, you burn extra calories and boost your overall metabolism. Not to mention its cholesterol-lowering effects.

Fresh flaxseed oil tastes great and enhances flavors, so it will help you enjoy your meals more! You can put the liquid form on almost anything, from your toast or steamed vegetables to pasta or baked potatoes. Think of it as melted butter or a delicious salad dressing.

My good friend, author of *Flax for Life!* and supplement expert Jade Beutler, says the addition of flax oil to your everyday diet is the single most important thing that you can do to positively impact your health and well-being. In fact, according to Jade your body is starving for good fat—the healthy fat called omega-3 that is abundant in flax oil. The health implications are profound as flax oil enhances optimal health and beauty from the inside out.

It is critically important that you chose only organic, high-quality, unfiltered, unrefined, refrigerated flax oil. Flaxseed oil is available in health food stores and some grocery stores, and you can also get it in capsule form.

NOTE: Visit JorgeCruise.com for links to my favorite brands.

Fruits

Fruits are just as beneficial as vegetables in terms of fiber and phytochemicals. But they contain a bit more sugar—and therefore, more calories—than vegetables. Regardless, you should enjoy these daily. To maximize your fat

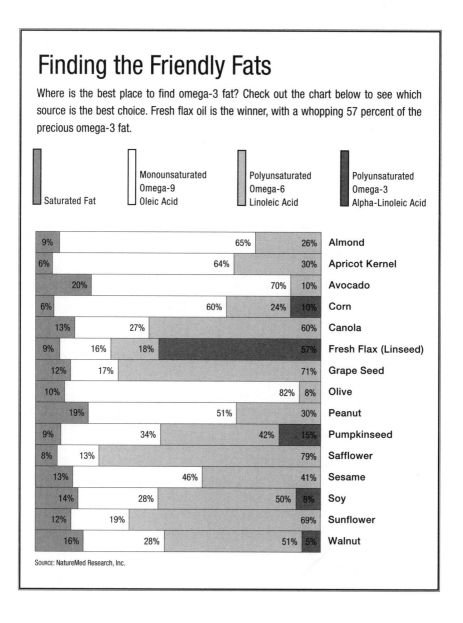

Finding the Friendly Fats

Where is the best place to find omega-3 fat? Check out the chart below to see which source is the best choice. Fresh flax oil is the winner, with a whopping 57 percent of the precious omega-3 fat.

Saturated Fat

Monounsaturated
Omega-9
Oleic Acid

Polyunsaturated
Omega-6
Linoleic Acid

Polyunsaturated
Omega-3
Alpha-Linoleic Acid

Saturated Fat	Oleic Acid	Linoleic Acid	Alpha-Linoleic Acid	
9%		65%	26%	Almond
6%		64%	30%	Apricot Kernel
20%		70%	10%	Avocado
6%		60%	24%	10%	Corn
13%	27%		60%	Canola
9%	16%	18%	57%	Fresh Flax (Linseed)
12%	17%		71%	Grape Seed
10%		82%	8%	Olive
19%		51%	30%	Peanut
9%	34%	42%	15%	Pumpkinseed
8%	13%		79%	Safflower
13%	46%		41%	Sesame
14%	28%	50%	8%	Soy
12%	19%		69%	Sunflower
16%	28%	51%	5%	Walnut

SOURCE: NatureMed Research, Inc.

burning, keep your fruit intake to one or two pieces a day, preferably with breakfast or as a snack.

Lemons and limes are the exception—you can use them as freely as your veggies. Eat vegetables at lunch and dinner. For a full list of recommended fruits and veggies, check out my 3-Hour Plate™ food lists in chapter 12.

Water

Although not a true food, water is essential for weight loss. More than half of your body is made up of water, and water helps keep nearly all of your bodily functions working smoothly and efficiently. Your kidneys need water to help filter toxins; your skin cells need water in order to stay plump and healthy; and your digestive tract needs water to flush out bodily waste.

Because it's filling and calorie-free, water is a dream come true when it comes to weight loss and maintenance. Water takes up room in your stomach, making you feel full. This means you'll eat less and feel less hungry. Of all the ways you can get fluid in your body, water is the best because it has zero calories. If you don't stick with plain water, your liquid calories can really add up. For example, a half-cup of fruit juice contains between 45 and 80 calories. So, at parties, keep a glass of water in your hand and sip it instead of grabbing a mixed drink—or any other type of drink, for that matter.

Finally, water also helps boost your metabolism by increasing your oxygen levels. A recent study completed in Germany found that drinking one 16-ounce glass of water boosts metabolism by 30 percent within forty minutes and keeps the metabolism elevated for more than an hour. According to this research, drinking eight 8-ounce glasses of water a day can burn off as many as 35,000 calories a year. That's 10 pounds of fat!

When you're dehydrated, you feel tired because your heart must work harder to pump your thirsty, thickened blood through your body. As a result, your muscles and organs don't get the oxygen and nutrients they need as quickly as they should.

Although many recommendations advise that you drink eight 8-ounce glasses of water a day, I suggest you drink at least half your body weight (in pounds) in ounces of water. If you weigh 160 pounds, aim for 80 ounces. Spread the water out by drinking one 10-ounce glass every hour for eight hours. By the time you get home at the end of the day, you'll have already drunk 80 ounces. This may sound daunting, but your body and waistline will thank you. Plus all the extra trips to the bathroom will increase your daily walking time!

My Favorite Water

To ensure you drink enough water every day, make sure you like the taste of the water you are drinking. Sometimes tap water leaves a chemical or mineral aftertaste. In that case, for cleaner tasting water you should switch to purified bottled water. I recommend Penta® ultrapremium purified drinking water; it's the purest bottled water I've found. It undergoes a 13-step, 11-hour purification process designed to remove every possible water impurity, including arsenic, bacteria, chlorine, chromium 6, fluoride, lead, MTBE, and pesticides. Penta®'s superclean, refreshing taste makes it easy to stay properly hydrated. Plus, Penta® acts as a superior detoxifier for your cells and improves cellular metabolism, helping you feel more invigorated and energized.

To make sure you're getting enough water, watch your urine. It should be light-colored or clear. If it's dark or strong-smelling, you're not drinking enough. Also watch for other signs of dehydration such as fatigue, headaches, and difficulty concentrating. And never depend on feeling thirsty to tell you when you need water. If you're thirsty, you're already dehydrated.

Here are some ways to ensure you get enough water:

- If you don't like the taste of plain water, try sparkling water such as Perrier®. Pour it in a glass and add a squeeze of lemon or lime.
- Drink a glass of water first thing in the morning. You may find that you no longer need your morning cup of coffee. One reason why many people feel tired in the morning is they are dehydrated!
- Drink a glass of water before every meal. Many people mistake thirst for hunger. Downing a glass of water will help you to stay in control of your eating and ensure you stick with the portions on your 3-Hour Plate™.

Choose your method of control

On the 3-Hour Diet™, you can choose from two simple visual methods of eating the right balance of foods at the right times:

1. You can follow the premade-meal plans in chapter 13.

2. You can follow my 3-Hour Plate™ system for custom meals.

Either way, you will be consuming approximately 1,450 calories a day, the right amount to help you shed 2 pounds of fat every week, but not so few calories that your body compensates by slowing your metabolism (see page 85). No matter whether you choose the 3-Hour Plate™ or the meal plans, you'll eat the correct balance of carbohydrates, proteins, and fats, which helps keep blood sugar and insulin levels in a normal range.

1) Using the Premade-Meal Plans

Broken into categories of breakfast, lunch/dinner, snacks, and treats in chapter 13, these meal plans are an easy way to stay on track. The meal plans work perfectly for people who want a premade blueprint to follow as they lose weight. Bottom line: the meal options will give you super-easy support to keep you on track—all with no deprivation and no calorie counting.

I've included meals you can cook at home, a number of frozen meals, and even fast-food options. I worked hard on these meals to make sure you would get the ideal balance of nutrients and the ideal amounts too. I've already figured out the best calorie content and mix of nutrients for you. All the work has been done for you. Each meal is perfectly *balanced* to give your body the right amount of carbohydrates, proteins, and fats that it needs. You can pick and choose the meals that interest you most. We have tested them all and they're all great. You can literally stick to your diet no matter where you find yourself—and no food is off-limits!

I suggest you plan your meals out at least the day before, by writing down what you will be eating each day for breakfast, lunch, and dinner on your 3-Hour Timeline™ found in chapter 9. Don't forget your snacks, treats, and water. These are just as important as your meals. **Assuming you weigh less than 200 pounds, you'll eat 400 calories at every meal, 100 calories for every snack, and 50 calories for your treats.** You'll find a list of great 100-calorie snacks and treats in chapter 13. If you weigh more than 200 pounds, you'll need to consume more food (see "The Right Number of Calories for Your Body"). Yes, you heard right. You will eat more if you are over 200 pounds to compensate for your body size.

Supplement Savvy

The growing interest in dietary and food supplements is also evident in all the media attention they receive. You practically can't turn on the TV without seeing an advertisement for a new supplement or hearing about studies of breakthrough supplements on the news. The following supplements are my favorites when it comes to helping you to lose weight.

FOOD SUPPLEMENT: FLAXSEED OIL

Why you need it: Of course, from reading pages 75–79 you known how much I love flax. Bottom line, flaxseed oil will help with the maintenance of your lean muscle tissue and thus help keep your resting metabolism strong. My recommendation to you is that you make this your fat of choice . . . not just a once in a while supplement. I use it each day with breakfast on my toast, at lunch on my salad as dressing and for dinner I use it on my dinner roll. Each serving should be 1 teaspoon or 4 capsules. Count it as your fat for that meal on your Cruise Timeline™.

FOOD SUPPLEMENT: GROUND FLAXSEED

Why you need it: I am also a fan of ground flaxseeds. The simple addition of ground flaxseeds to your daily diet will result in the removal of belly bulge. Yep think about it . . . a flatter belly. How does this work? Ground flaxseed is an excellent source of both soluble and insoluble dietary *fiber* which will cleanse the intestinal tract and regulate elimination. All this helps to remove extra internal belly bulge. Yep you would be surprised how much of your belly bulge is not fat, but rather fecal matter that is stuck from a low fiber diet. Plus once ingested ground flax binds to simple sugars and carbohydrates slowing their release into the blood stream. The result is enhanced levels of energy and endurance between your 3-hour meals.

SUPPLEMENT: WHEY PROTEIN POWDER

Why you need them: When it comes to supplemental forms of protein to maximize your retention of fat burning lean muscle tissue, whey protein is the best. Whey protein has the highest bio-absorption levels. This means your body's muscles will stay more structurally supported and thus your metabolism revved. I love a chocolate scoop of whey protein powder blended in water with ice as a delicious 100 calorie snack drink.

SUPPLEMENT: VITAMIN C POWDER

Why you need it: Vitamin C is a dietary antioxidant that helps to eliminate free radical damage in and around your cells including your lean muscle fibers. Bottom line, vitamin C helps minimize damage to your tissues, helps with the rebuilding of new muscle and even keeps your immune system strong. The best form to take vitamin C in is powder form with a glass of water since it will absorb into your system more efficiently. I take it every day—ideally 1,000 milligrams.

FOOD SUPPLEMENT: GREENS SUPER FOODS

Why you need it: Greens Super Foods help reduce appetite between meals. How? Greens Super Foods are one of the richest sources of naturally occurring vitamins, minerals, and phyto-nutrients. This super rich source helps curb the appetite by providing the body a high, nutrient dense food source. Yep, you see the more dense in nutrients a food is the more satiated you will feel. And as a bonus, the micro-algae chlorella closely resembles the oxygen-carrying component of the red blood cell called hemoglobin. As a result, chlorella enhances the ability for the body to use oxygen, increasing energy and endurance.

SUPPLEMENT: MULTI-VITAMIN

Why you need it: In the 3-hour diet there are no banned foods, and at the same time we want to ensure that your bodies nutritional needs are fully met so you are not left feeling hungry or craving high calorie, low quality foods between meals. Taking a complete multivitamin/mineral enables you to fulfill your body's nutrient barometer—turning off the instinct to consume excess calories.

SUPPLEMENT: GREEN TEA

Why you need it: What if there was a nutritional superstar that possessed all of the benefits of a stimulant in enhancing metabolism, but without any of the negative consequences? Well, it is green tea. Green tea contains naturally occurring caffeine. However, unlike caffeine or the now banned ephedra—caffeine in green tea does not negatively effect the body—but does increase metabolism, caloric burning, and weight loss.

NOTE: Visit JorgeCruise.com for links to my favorite brands.

THE RIGHT NUMBER OF CALORIES FOR YOUR BODY

Whether you choose my premade meals or create your own custom 3-Hour Plate™ meals, you will consume roughly 1,450 calories a day. Although I've done all of the calorie counting for you, I thought you'd like to see how those calories break down into meals and snacks.

MEAL 1: Breakfast	400 calories of balanced nutrients
MEAL 2: Snack A	100 calories
MEAL 3: Lunch	400 calories of balanced nutrients
MEAL 4: Snack B	100 calories
MEAL 5: Dinner	400 calories of balanced nutrients
MEAL 6: Treat	50 calories

NOTE: Depending on your current weight, you may need to adjust this plan to your personal metabolism. Assuming you weigh less than 200 pounds, the above plan will work for you. However, if you weigh more, make the following changes:

200 to 249 pounds: double your snack size to 200 calories
250 to 299 pounds: triple your snack size to 300 calories
300 pounds or more: quadruple your snack size to 400 calories or add another meal

As your weight drops, move to the next calorie selection to continue losing 2 pounds a week.

If you weigh less than 150 pounds and are short in stature (under 5'3"), 1,450 calories may be too much food for you. You can solve this simply by cutting your breakfast in half and eating only 200 calories during this meal, for a total intake of 1,250 calories. See page 258 for more details.

2) Using the Visual 3-Hour Plate™

If you'd like more freedom to choose what you eat rather than use my premade-meal plans, you can follow my 3-Hour Plate™. This simple eating plan will help you automatically eat the right foods in the right portions so you turn down your appetite and turn up your fat-burning furnace.

Each part of the 3-Hour Plate™ performs a distinct function for overall health and weight loss. The 3-Hour Plate™ will also allow you to eat the foods you love while adding a few crucial foods to help slow down your appetite and speed up your metabolism.

For example, you might eat a high fiber cereal with almonds and one half of a grapefruit for breakfast, vegetable soup and a sandwich of reduced-

HOW TO ESTIMATE
PORTION SIZES

1 cup	=	1 fist or a baseball
⅓ cup	=	1 cupped hand (palm)
½ cup of cut fruit, cooked vegetables	=	1 rounded handful or small fist
3 ounces of meat, poultry, or fish	=	1 women's palm
1 piece of fruit	=	a light bulb
1 teaspoon	=	1 thumb tip (tip of thumb to knuckle)
1 tablespoon	=	3 thumb tips
2 tablespoons of peanut butter	=	a ping pong or golf ball
1 ounce of cheese	=	1 thumb
1 ounce of nuts	=	1 cupped palmful
2 ounces of chips or pretzels	=	2 cupped palmfuls
6 ounces of chicken breast	=	1 fist
3 oz. cooked meat	=	a deck of cards
4 ounces of fish	=	1 cupped hand
1 ounce bread or grain	=	a cassette tape
1 serving broccoli	=	a light bulb
1 medium potato	=	a computer mouse or cassette tape

calorie bread, turkey, lean bacon, and avocado for lunch, and a taco filled with lean meat plus a mixed green salad for dinner. (For a detailed list of food suggestions and portion sizes for your meals, see chapter 12.)

You'll notice that the protein portion of the plate contains three divisions. You can either fill those slots with one 3-ounce serving of protein (a total roughly the size of a deck of cards), or two to three different, smaller servings. For example, instead of having a plain 3-ounce chicken breast, you can have a 2-ounce piece of chicken smothered with 1 ounce of cheese.

Whether you follow the all-new 3-Hour Plate™ or use the premade-meal plans, *timing is everything*. Starting with breakfast (yes, breakfast is extremely important!), you must eat every 3 hours. Follow these pointers:

1. To get your metabolism revving, eat your first meal within an hour of getting out of bed. If you don't eat within that first

The 3-Hour Plate™

How it works: For breakfast, lunch, and dinner, use a standard 9-inch dinner plate and fill half the plate with vegetables (fruit is recommended for breakfast) the equivalent of three DVD cases. Then mentally divide the other half into two parts and fill the remainder of the plate with carbohydrates the equivalent of a Rubik's Cube®, protein the equivalent of a deck of playing cards, and then also include a teaspoon of fat to help curb your appetite the equivalent of a water bottle cap. If you're still hungry after finishing the plate, you can add another plate of veggies or fruit, equivalent to 3 DVD cases. It's that simple!

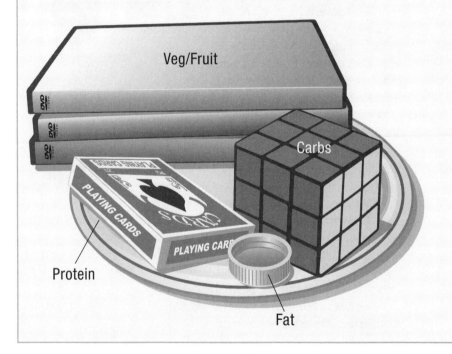

crucial hour, your body will turn down your metabolism to try to hold on to the calorie-rich tissue in your body. And many of my clients also just forget to eat if they don't make a conscious effort to eat within that first hour upon waking.

2. After breakfast, eat five more times (for a total of six) throughout the day, separated by 3 hours. You might eat breakfast at 7 a.m.,

Height: 5'2"
Age: 46
Starting weight: 174 lbs.
Current weight: 134 lbs.
Other: A self-employed mother of 3
  grown children, grandmother of 1; lives
  with her boyfriend, daughter, 2 dogs,
  turtle, and lovebird

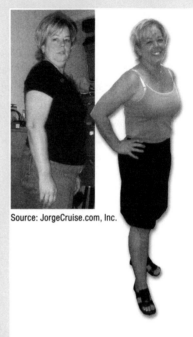

Source: JorgeCruise.com, Inc.

"I've wanted to lose weight for a long time. When I looked in the mirror, I did not see a person I liked. I hated looking at photos of myself, and was embarrassed when others saw them. I kept buying new clothes, always a size larger than before. It was horrible.

"I went to the doctor for a physical. She referred me to a weight-loss clinic that promotes a liquid diet. I didn't want to use a drink to get in shape, so I decided to try Jorge's 3-Hour Diet™ instead. Now, even though I have not met my goal weight, I see a slimmer person. I feel much more in control of my destiny.

"**This diet has changed my life.** I have a little more spunk in my step, I feel better, I sleep better, and I am fitting into smaller clothes. My coworkers have noticed, too. I am much happier than I used to be. Stress at work used to make me break down and cry; now I can handle it. It's no big deal. When I was not eating right, it affected my whole life negatively. Now, I eat all the time, and am loving it.

"I look forward to continuing my weight loss, and using the knowledge I have learned regarding food with Jorge to help others."

Annette's Secrets to Success

- ➤ Clip a kitchen timer to your clothing. Set it to beep every three hours to remind you to eat.
- ➤ Look at all the smaller clothes in your closet that no longer fit—but one day will.

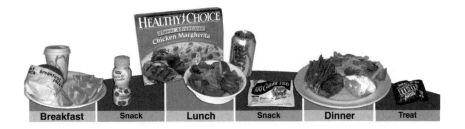

then have one of your snacks at 10 a.m., eat lunch at 1 p.m.,
have another snack at 4 p.m., and dinner at 7 p.m. with a treat
shortly thereafter. This is a perfect eating schedule, and I suggest
you follow it as closely as you can.

3. Your treat can be enjoyed with your dinner or 3 hours after
   dinner, whatever you prefer. The treat is only 50 calories, so if
   you do decide to eat it 3 hours after dinner, you don't have to
   wait 3 hours to go to bed.

Critical in the 3-Hour Diet™ are the snacks and treats. These pit stops
will help fuel your metabolism all day long, allowing you to eat small bits
of food every three hours and nurture your body with regular doses of calories that will rev up fat burning. You'll eat a snack mid-morning and mid-
afternoon, and a delicious treat after dinner. Each snack should total about
100 calories (two a day) and each treat about 50 calories. I've included a list
of great snacks and treats in chapter 13.

Point 3: The magic of preparation

Some people ask me how I can eat certain vegetables, such as broccoli
or spinach. They tell me they hate these foods. I tell them the magic is in
the preparation. You can make just about any foods taste wonderful by
adding herbs and spices. Experiment with garlic, cilantro, basil, and
other fresh herbs. Mix in some sautéed onion. If you like spicy foods, try
sprinkling on a Cajun spice blend. Experiment and find the mix that's
right for you. Most foods taste fantastic when you add a simple mixture
of olive oil, rice vinegar, salt, and pepper. Take one part each of oil and

vinegar and add salt and pepper to taste. Mix it all up and taste. You'll love it!

Chef Bernard, my good friend, member of my advisory circle, and award-winning chef, says "A good cook is a sorcerer who dispenses happiness on a plate." I agree. Below are some secrets that he has shared with me on how to be a good sorcerer in the kitchen.

Vegetables

- Freshness is the key. It is important to choose a good variety daily.
- Never refrigerate tomatoes!!!! For best flavor store at room temperature and use when fully ripened, but still firm.
- Maintain the integrity of the ingredients' taste by using simple cooking techniques such as stir frying and grilling.
- Jazz it up with you favorite herbs, spices, or citrus zest.
- Steam vegetables rapidly with a limited amount of water; it will prevent a loss of the precious nutrients.

Poultry

- Prior to cooking poultry, wash and pat dry!
- When roasting chicken on a rack, place aromatic herbs and [sun-dried fruit] under the skin. It will infuse the meat.
- Let roasted chicken rest for 10 to 15 minutes before carving to allow juices to be distributed throughout the meat.
- Grilling a bone-in chicken breast and leaving the skin on will help to hold in juices, which increases tenderness.
- When frying or browning chicken in a pan, use a nonstick skillet, which requires less added fat and enhance the flavor with a ginger citrus marinade.
- Use a meat thermometer to ensure that the meat is fully cooked. The thermometer should read 170° when inserted into the thickest part of the thigh and 165° when inserted into the breast.

Red meat

- Choose the highest grade quality of beef to enjoy the deepest flavor.
- The most tender cuts of beef are obtained from the center of the animal, such as the loin and rib area.

- Cooking a bone-in beef steak using a high-temperature cooking method will seal in natural juices, so leave the grill uncovered.
- Cut large pieces of meat into 2-inch portions before marinating. Thinner cuts of meat marinate more quickly and will create the perfect size for kabobs.
- When cooking a marinated flank steak, baste meats during the last 5-10 minutes of grilling to maximize flavor.

Seafood

- Look for local, natural products and do not be afraid to experiment with different varieties.
- The best fish for grilling tends to be a meatier fish such as salmon, halibut, swordfish, tuna, or sea bass.
- Boil shrimp, lobster, or crab in an aromatic broth to showcase their delicate flavors.
- To retain the moisture during the cooking process, pan-sear your fish fillet with the skin on.
- Create a different sensation of taste and texture by coating fish with fresh herbs, nuts, or spices.

Dessert

- Every day, stop by the market and select your favorite seasonal fresh fruits and berries.
- Phyllo dough is a great substitute for a spiced apricot turnover.

Bottom line: Chef Bernard's best advice for preparation is to experiment and find the mix that's right for you.

How to make it super tempting

Now you know everything you need to know in order to be super-successful. And with what we learned in chapter 5, you now have both secrets in your hand.

Before you do, however, I want you to do a little exercise that will help you to dive into the 3-Hour Diet™ with greater gusto. This exercise will help you to feel even more drawn to the diet. Rather than feel as if you must push yourself to stick with the diet, you'll feel pulled to it.

My Ten Favorite Foods

List your ten favorite foods here:

1. _____

2. _____

3. _____

4. _____

5. _____

6. _____

7. _____

8. _____

9. _____

10. _____

P.S. Photocopy this list and place it on your refrigerator.

The only way you can feel strongly drawn is if it contains your favorite foods. You can only look forward to eating if you will be eating foods you really love. It's that simple. So what I want you to do right now is turn to the food lists in Chapter 12. Take a look at the carbohydrate, protein, fat, and other food options. Look at the meal plans in Chapter 13. Then in the space above write down ten foods or meal ideas from those examples that you really love. These should be foods and meals that make your mouth water when you think about them. They should be your favorite foods of all time.

Then, once you've done that, you're ready to take action. Remember, by eliminating banned foods, you will be able to eat absolutely anywhere, from parties to buffets to family dinners. You will have the freedom to enjoy the foods you love (even fast food), and you will gain the self-confidence that comes from knowing you have the power to control the foods you eat.

PART III

Overcoming Obstacles

SEVEN

HOW TO MAKE MORE TIME

ix months ago my doctor expressed concern over the results from my physical. I had become borderline everything and he suggested all sorts of medicine, which wouldn't have been good for my liver. All the medical problems that surfaced from that physical were a direct result of being overweight. Before I started the program, I would get exhausted sweeping our kitchen floor, and was taking medicine for my high blood pressure. Today, I no longer take blood pressure medicine and I have enough energy to complete any task I start. I am able to hike seven to ten miles and can carry around forty-five pounds in my pack. My more physical friends now invite me on their outings—we have made plans to hike with friends in Nevada next spring."

—JOSÉ COLÓN—LOST 54 POUNDS

If your day feels like a race from the moment you get out of bed until the moment you lie back down, you might be thinking that you might not have time to regularly eat every three hours.

Lack of time can be a concern. In fact, it can be the top reason more people stop dieting and exercising. Yet it doesn't have to be this way, at least not for you. As you will soon discover, you have more time than you think. Here's the great thing I have learned from working with over three million online clients: we all have exactly 24 hours a day to live our lives. Whether you are Oprah Winfrey, the president of the United States, a business executive, or a stay-at-home mom, you have just as much time as anyone else.

So the real question you must ask yourself isn't "Where am I going to find the time?" It's "How will I stay committed to this?" In this chapter, you will discover and build your commitment in a two-step process:

1. Identify your Loser Zones: the places where you waste time rather than make it
2. Discover an emotional spark that reinforces your commitment

The good news is that you'll soon learn you indeed have time. You just have to commit yourself to making it. You really can do it.

I will show you how. The secret is to manage your time better and not lose it. You DO have the time; you just might not know it yet.

Not only will you discover the lost time you desperately need to dedicate to your healthy eating, but you will also experience a deep feeling of freedom and higher self-esteem. You will glow from knowing you have made yourself a top priority. If you are a parent, you will feel like a better parent knowing you have become a "healthier" role model for your kids.

Discover Your Loser Zones

All of us have what I call a Loser Zone, a zone where we spend too much time on things that don't really matter to us. You're in a Loser Zone when you spend time doing something that makes no significant improvement in your life. The #1 Loser Zone activity is watching television. The average American spends 30 hours a week in front of the tube. Surfing the Internet and aimlessly chatting on the phone also rank high as Loser Zone activities. My clients with poor time management skills usually have no idea how long their daily tasks take them to complete.

Step back and take a good hard look at how you spend your time. Keep

My Loser Zones

Loser Zone 1: _____

Hours per day: _____

Loser Zone 2: _____

Hours per day: _____

Loser Zone 3: _____

Hours per day: _____

Total number of hours today:

This is your *newfound* time to prepare and/or eat your meals.

track of everything you do and how much time you spend doing it, for three days in a row. Yes, you must actually watch the time by looking at your watch right before and right after you do something. You may be surprised at how much time certain tasks actually take you to complete. Maybe you spend 30 percent of your time at work, 5 percent of your time driving, 5 percent getting ready to leave the house, 5 percent talking on the phone, 10 percent cleaning, and so on. After you've mapped out your time, realistically assess whether you are allocating your time wisely.

Once you've created your log, I want you to take a good hard look at it and pick three Loser Zone activities that you could do without. Write them down in the space provided. Then, write down how much time you spend on average in each Loser Zone, each day. Finally, add up your zones. This total is the number of hours you can create each day for the 3-Hour Diet™ simply by eliminating your Loser Zones.

The Jorge Cruise Time Management System

Now that you have discovered more time to spend on the 3-Hour Diet™, it's time to cement your commitment to the program. If you don't create a reason that resonates deep inside for why you want to spend time doing the 3-Hour Diet™, you'll never spend time doing the 3-Hour Diet™. It's that simple.

To build that commitment, you must focus on the positive reasons to lose weight. Too often, people focus on the negative—on the weight. I've learned over the years that you get what you focus on. So when you focus in on being fat, you end up getting fatter. You must instead focus on getting thinner—and on all of the positive reasons that motivate you to get and stay thin. I have learned over the years that the people who are most successful at losing weight are the ones who focus on why they want to lose the weight. They tell me they want to go to Egypt and climb the Pyramids, or take a vacation in the Caribbean and feel confident when wearing a bathing suit. They keep their eyes on a target in the future and aim themselves toward that target.

You will now learn to do the same with this three-step time management process:

- Pinpoint your targets
- Make an emotional connection to your targets
- Lock in your targets

Pinpoint your targets

What are the reasons you want to lose weight? Of course you want to look good—but *why*? Maybe you want to lose weight because you feel it will help you to meet your life partner. Perhaps losing weight will allow you to accomplish a life dream, such as climbing to the top of a mountain. Maybe you want to lose weight because it will give you the energy you need to play all day with your kids. Perhaps you want to look good at an upcoming event, such as a wedding or high school reunion.

Come up with three to ten targets. These targets should not be about losing weight on the scale or about burning fat. They should be things that make you emotional: things that touch your heart and fire you up about losing the weight. Make sure some of your targets are long-term. It's fine to write a few short-term targets such as looking great for a specific event, but you should have some long-term ones as well, such as getting healthy so you can play with your children—and grandchildren.

Make an emotional connection to your targets

Now it's time to look a little deeper. It's time to really examine those targets and uncover your deepest motivation for achieving them.

If you are emotional about something, you are going to do it. I will always remember when my dad was diagnosed with prostate cancer. For

My Targets

1. _____

2. _____

3. _____

4. _____

5. _____

6. _____

7. _____

8. _____

9. _____

10. _____

Why I Want to Accomplish Them

_____
_____
_____

_____
_____
_____

_____
_____
_____

_____
_____
_____

_____
_____
_____

_____
_____
_____

_____
_____
_____

_____
_____
_____

_____
_____
_____

_____
_____
_____

years he hadn't cared about healthy eating or exercising. He said he didn't have time. But once he was diagnosed with cancer, and his doctor told him he had just a year to live, my dad suddenly found the time to eat right and exercise. It was effortless for him. Did he find a twenty-fifth or twenty-sixth hour in the day to spend on his weight loss efforts? Of course not. He just changed his priorities and got motivated.

Now it's time for you to do the same. Ask yourself "How will this target improve my life?" For example, if you chose the target "have more energy for my children", that target might improve your life by making life more fulfilling, giving you a sense of pride, and drawing you closer to your family. If you want to look good in a swim suit on vacation, that target might allow you to do some things you've never done before, such as swim with dolphins in the ocean or hang out at the hotel pool with your family.

For each of your targets, I now want you to list three deep emotional reasons why you want to accomplish them in the space provided.

Lock in your targets

Now that you have created some pretty motivational reasons to lose weight, it's time to use those reasons not only to commit to the program, but to commit to creating time for the program. You will do this by locking yourself in: by scheduling time for the program. Use the Cruise Timeline™ from chapter 5 and commit yourself to eating every 3 hours. Write down your meals and the times you are going to eat them. You now have now discovered the time to do so and the motivation to do so—so get to it!

Change Your Attitude

Before we end this chapter, I want to make sure you are aware that a large part of success on the 3-Hour Diet™—and life in general—is attitude. Yep. I've heard that attitude is half the battle; I'd say it's more than that. You may get some useful tips from my program, but the real secret lies inside of you! If you bring forth the maximum amount of emotion inside of you, you will move forward much more quickly. Your outlook, your willingness to learn, and your perspective on life will play a large part in your results.

Many of us have developed bad habits, and frankly, bad attitudes that have to be broken. To start breaking out of unhealthy, unproductive patterns, ask yourself: Why do I do things this way? Would I get better results if I did them differently?

Height: 5"3'
Age: 45
Start weight: 273 lbs.
Current weight: 186 lbs.
Other: Mother of a 21-year-old
    son in college; general
    manager of a retail store

"Before I saw Jorge on the news one morning, I was not really living. I went to work and came home. I didn't want to go anywhere because someone might see that I was fat. At home and at work, I felt safe because everyone there already knew. I tried to erase myself from everyone's memories, too. I would not allow my picture to be taken and I wouldn't join any family events. I never had much energy, and I never had any mirrors around. I didn't fit in any clothes correctly and I was eating secretly and emotionally.

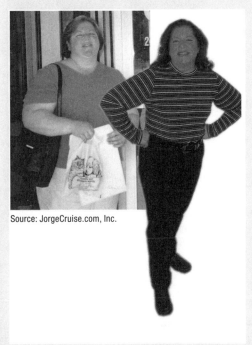

Source: JorgeCruise.com, Inc.

"Each Monday, I planned to start a new diet. I would eat anything I wanted on Saturday and Sunday in anticipation. The problem was Monday rarely ever came, but there were lots of Saturdays and Sundays. Pretty soon I saw I was pushing 300 pounds. I became a vegetarian in January 2004 and gained even more weight.

"Something Jorge said that morning really struck me, and I have followed his directions to a "T". I want to help other people do the same. Everything he says makes sense. His plan is so easy to follow. **I do not hide from mirrors any longer and I feel great.**

"If you commit to this and follow the plan you will succeed. I will 'fuel' myself like this forever."

SUSAN'S SECRETS TO SUCCESS
Prepare & Portion!

On Sunday mornings I do my shopping for the week. I go to Windmill Farms, Whole Foods, and Costco. I also go to Smart & Final to purchase all of my portion cups.

That afternoon I prepare the food and portion it out into cups for the week. *Nothing* stays in its original container or package. I realized early on that I cannot portion as I go because I do not measure correctly and I would often skip a meal if I didn't prepare ahead. I make sure I prepare and portion out enough meals and snacks for the whole week. You can see by the pictures that I am well prepared for the week ahead with no chance of cheating or skipping.

At work and throughout my day, I have a five-alarm watch that is preset for 6 a.m., 9 a.m., 12 p.m., 3 p.m., and 6 p.m. I plan *all* events around my eating schedule. Even if I am in a meeting and my alarm goes off, I eat no matter what. I decided that the 3-Hour Diet™ comes first. My boss understands and my employees even help me to remember. If my alarm goes off and I am not at my desk, someone on the sales floor will yell, "Snack time!"

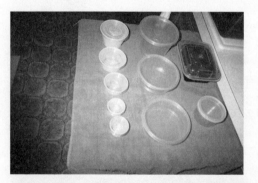

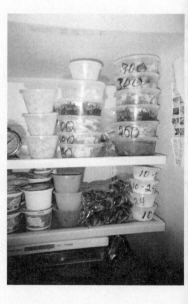

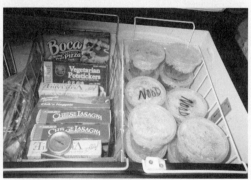

Secrets to Locking In Your Targets

To stay on track on your 3-Hour Diet™, you need to do prioritize your tasks and do the right thing at the right time. Here's how:

Maximize the first two hours of your day. For most of us, the first two hours of the day are when we're filled with the most energy and enthusiasm. Make the most of this productive time. Fit as many of the tasks on your daily to-do list into these two hours as you can. Not only will you get things done, you'll also be able to spend the rest of your day with a sense of accomplishment.

Do your most unpleasant tasks first. You will never dislike an unpleasant task any less if you put it off. It's human nature to procrastinate, especially when it comes to tasks like cleaning out the fridge or getting your oil changed. So get these things over with. Then you'll be left with the rest of your day to do things you enjoy.

Give yourself a break. Now and then you're not going to get to every single thing on your to-do list or follow the 3-Hour Diet™ to a "T". Your to-do list should act as a "best-case scenario" for your life. You and I both know that not all days go so smoothly, so forgive yourself if you stray slightly from your schedule—you'll get back on track the next day. The worst thing you can do is allow yourself to feel guilty. Guilty feelings will only waste valuable time and energy you could be storing up to finish all your tasks the next day. Plus, they can lead you to overeat.

Stay on track. Most of us can identify with this scenario: You set aside a Saturday to clean out your attic. While sifting through some boxes, you come across an old photo album and spend more than an hour flipping through its pages. Then you come across another album. At the end of the day you've only cleaned out a small part of the attic!

To avoid this kind of time trap, stay focused on the task at hand. If your goal is to clean your attic, then clean your attic. Avoid the temptation to dive into old albums or try on old clothes. This piece of advice can be utilized in all areas of your life, from your workplace to your kitchen.

Whether you're packing your snacks for the next day or ironing your clothes, stay on task. Don't become distracted by what's in the fridge and start making a grocery list, or start sifting through your closet and cleaning out what you don't need. Just keep packing or ironing and write yourself a note to remind yourself to tackle the other chores when you have some spare time.

Height: 5'3"
Age: 25
Starting Weight: 131 lbs.
Current Weight: 118 lbs.
Other: Works full time (12- to 14-hour days); very little free time

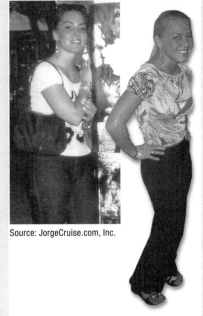

Source: JorgeCruise.com, Inc.

"Before Jorge Cruise, I saw a heavy, struggling, tired person. Someone who exercises but many times ate too much (and knew it), snacked too often, and craved sugar all the time. I always thought I had a pretty face, but was consistently disappointed with the way pants fit, with my face in photos, my thighs in general, and always the size of my calves.

"To feel the way I feel now is incredible. The biggest critic in my life has always been my mother; this is according to me—in my mind. I have always noticed what she says and thinks. However, I would hope and assume that my mom would love me whether I weighed 200 pounds or 110 pounds. Like me, my mom has always worried about her weight even though she is 54, has had four children, works as a nurse in a hospital, exercises, and weighs 128 pounds. **Well, I saw my mom on my birthday a couple months ago and she said I looked 'good.' A month went by until I saw her again and she exclaimed, 'You look so skinny!' Well, those words meant a lot—in fact, more than my size 4 jeans feeling loose.**

"I understand that 'skinny' may not be the healthiest word but it sure felt good. My mom's comment and many other people's comments only motivate me to further my efforts in maintaining my weight and commitment to sticking to Jorge's great, easy, explainable 3-hour plan. Not only can I explain why the plan works to myself but to others as well—it is a livable plan."

Claire's Secrets to Success

- ➤ PLAN! PLAN! PLAN!
- ➤ If you have a hectic schedule such as my own, have lots of Pria bars, almonds, fruit, and other easy-to-eat items close at hand.
- ➤ I try to eat before I go out or go shopping so I am not starving when I order or arrive, and then eat the wrong thing or too much.

To start to change your attitude, engage in the following practices:

Surround yourself with successful people. If you spend time with people you respect and admire, you will start to emulate their behaviors, consciously or subconsciously. Their enthusiasm will rub off on you. While out for dinner with your fit, slim friend Sarah, you'll be inspired to adopt her ways and you too will order the grilled vegetable plate. If you go out for dinner with an overweight friend who orders a creamy alcoholic drink and a four course meal, you'll be tempted to do the same. This is not to say that you shouldn't spend any time with friends whose habits you don't admire; just wisely choose the situations in which you socialize with them. A great place to meet thousands of people who are committed to getting and staying healthy is our JorgeCruise.com Web site club. Make sure to visit it, connect, and meet new buddies.

Expand your horizons. Instead of dismissing a novel activity because you don't know what to expect, jump right in! Seek out new ways to challenge yourself and stop being afraid to take chances. Once you step out of your comfort zone, you'll realize there's a whole new world out there for you.

Don't fear failure. Every person who has achieved success—myself included—has failed at some point along the way. If you haven't failed, you haven't tried hard enough. The secret is being able to look at failure as an opportunity for learning, as a chance to reflect on what went wrong and what you can do to improve your results next time.

Take responsibility for your actions. If you don't feel accountable for the way you conduct yourself, what's stopping you from shirking your responsibilities? Keep promises you make to your friends and family. Make your deadlines. If you say you're going to meet your friend for lunch at a certain time, be there and be there on time. The more you get in the habit of keeping your promises to others, the more you'll keep your promises to yourself.

Do the best you can. Each of us is born with a unique set of talents, personality traits, and quirks. You know yourself better than anyone in the world and you know when you've put your best foot forward. And that's all you can do. When you've worked as hard as you can, congratulate yourself and celebrate!

Meal Options for Busy People

When I was testing and creating the 3-Hour Diet™ thousands of my online clients requested that I create extra convenient ways to live the 3-Hour Diet™. Literally ways that would give them more time by freeing them completely from meal preparation. Ways that would take absolutely no effort. So I am thrilled to share with you our meal options for busy people on the go:

1. Fresh-delivered meals. Imagine receiving three delicious 400-calorie gourmet meals, two 100-calorie snacks, and one treat delivered fresh to your door each day.
2. Meal bars and shakes. Imagine carrying within your purse, briefcase, or anywhere a perfect nutritionally balanced 400-calorie meal in one delicious bar or shake.
3. Snack bars. For between meals you could indulge in a delicious 100-calorie snack bar that will keep your metabolism going strong.

Visit JorgeCruise.com/meals for more details.

EIGHT

OVERCOMING EMOTIONAL EATING

"A few years ago, a tragedy in our family caused me to gain over 60 pounds within one year. When I looked in the mirror, all I saw was a hopeless situation. My routine used to be a fruit shake in the morning and a diet shake for lunch. I was so hungry by the time I got home that I would eat whatever food was within reach—with no regard to calories or nutritional value. I heard Jorge on television talking about the 3-Hour Diet™. His plan made sense to me and I was excited to get started. My favorite thing about this lifestyle, besides watching the weight disappear, is how simple it is to follow."

—VICKIE FREY—LOST 22 POUNDS

Before she came to see me, Sarah used to think about food constantly. When she wasn't eating, she was daydreaming about what she would cook for her next meal, or brainstorming restaurants to hit for lunch. A few hours after dinner, she would plop down in front of the television with a box of cookies or bag of microwave popcorn and finish the whole thing without thinking twice.

After I talked with Sarah, I learned she had been divorced a few years earlier. Her husband moved out of her life and food moved in, putting more than 50 extra pounds on her body and squashing the potential for any new relationships—with all her thoughts about eating, she simply didn't have the time.

Sarah was a classic emotional eater. Instead of facing the pain she felt over losing her husband, she quelled that pain with food. To compensate, she often skipped breakfast and tried to eat as little as possible for lunch. After she arrived home from work, however, she was famished—and the eating began with reckless abandon.

Thankfully, Sarah started the 3-Hour Diet™. She gained control of her emotional eating and learned to fill her emotional holes with what she needed—human attention and nurturing.

The Hungry Heart

Can you identify with Sarah's struggle? Have you ever overeaten when you weren't hungry? Have you ever turned to french fries or ice cream to fill a void or numb pain? Has food ever made you feel supported or comforted?

When you eat when you're not hungry, chances are you're eating for emotional reasons. Emotional eating is only a symptom of a much larger problem, a hurtful void or emptiness in your life. It's not your stomach that's hungry—it's your heart. Emotional eating is the #1 saboteur of all diets.

It's no surprise so many people use food as a crutch. Life can be stressful. Some of my clients recall being sexually abused and then turning to food to numb the pain and hide their bodies. Other people eat out of loneliness, boredom, or sadness.

If you are an emotional eater, you have to make a new choice. To successfully lose weight, you must stop using food as a crutch to quell your emotions. You must find a better kind of emotional support, something that won't widen your waistline.

To overcome emotional eating, you must first learn to discern between emotional hunger and nutritional hunger. Nutritional hunger is a biological need—we need the calories, vitamins, and minerals that come from food to stay healthy and build lean muscle. Emotional hunger, on the other hand, comes from a lack of warmth, support, and companionship from other people. To step off the emotional eating roller coaster, you must start to feed your emotional needs with support from friends and family.

When you overcome emotional eating, you will

1. **Achieve true freedom long-term.** As an emotional eater, you are hindering your freedom to enjoy eating. Instead of taking pleasure in a piece of cake to celebrate a positive life event such as a birthday or graduation, you use sweets to numb something negative that happened in your past. Overcoming emotional eating will give you the freedom to enjoy parties and celebrations—all joyous events that involve food.
2. **Stop the self-sabotage.** By ceasing to eat for emotional reasons, you will no longer use food as a barrier between you and your emotions. You will be forced to deal with the issues at hand instead of drowning them with chocolate sauce and milkshakes. When you look face-to-face at the issues fueling your emotional eating, you can begin to take the steps necessary to resolve them. You will become a more empowered, stronger you.
3. **Stop being enslaved by food.** You may feel as if you're trapped behind walls of potato chips, cookies, and french fries, and the only way to get out of your prison is to eat your way through. This is all in your mind. If you look for friendship and support in the right places, you'll find people who will tear down those food walls and give you the non-food comfort you crave!

When you break out of your food prison, food will become a source of pleasure in your life once again, a pleasure you can control. Instead of calling your name in the middle of the night, your favorite dessert will be a treat, a way you reward yourself for a full day of good eating behavior.

What Is Emotional Eating?

As I suggested above, you engage in emotional eating when you're hungry for things other than food. You think you're craving a chocolate chip cheesecake, when actually you crave emotional comfort and support. There is a hurtful void or emptiness in your life that you can't seem to fill, so you fill it with food.

Human beings are hardwired to avoid pain and seek out pleasure. You enjoy eating the cheesecake because it takes your mind off your sadness,

The 3-Hour Solution

Overcoming emotional eating will help you to

- Achieve true freedom long term
- Stop the self-sabotage
- Stop being enslaved by food

and it makes you feel better. Food becomes your best friend, your #1 comforter, and your supporter. You fill your stomach to fill your void. But emotional eating is like trying to fill a hole in the desert with water. Once the water seeps in or the food is digested, you're left with the same hole that was there before. All you've done is gain calories and fat.

My good friend and the emotional-eating expert on my advisory circle, Linda Spangle, the author of *Life is Hard, Food is Easy* says, "With emotional eating, food is the 'consolation prize'—better than nothing, but not even close to what you really wanted, such as love, appreciation, or nurturing. To stop these destructive patterns that contribute to overeating, you need to learn new ways to fill your heart."

The pattern goes like this: You have a defining event or events in your life that left you emotionally scarred. You don't get the nurturing, love, or support you need to heal that scar; instead, you have a painful thorn. This thorn continues to pierce you, leaving you with emptiness, distress, and pain. If you don't get the emotional support you need to yank the thorn out, you're likely to turn to something that numbs the pain. Food numbs you, at least while you're eating it, so you become addicted to food and—surprise, you gain weight.

The good news: You can stop this vicious cycle. Just follow my 3-step plan.

Step 1: Accept yourself

In order to lose weight, you must first learn to love your body. Your body is the greatest gift you will ever receive. It's an astonishing machine that does

Height: 5'5"
Age: 47
Starting weight: 235 lbs.
Current weight: 165 lbs.
Other: A single mom with 2
   grown children; works full
   time

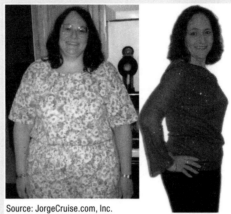

Source: JorgeCruise.com, Inc.

"Before the 3-Hour Diet™, I was miserable. I had given up any hope of losing weight. I had failed every diet I had tried, and gained back the weight that was lost plus more!

"I was an overweight child, an overweight teenager, and an overweight adult. My weight continued to climb through two pregnancies and a divorce. At the age of 30, I was diagnosed with lupus. My medication not only caused me to gain 50 more pounds but made my body and face look bloated. I looked like a balloon. Also, because I was so sick I had to quit my job and go on welfare. Very depressing!

"After a few years when my lupus was under control, I was able to go back to work. I weighed in at 260 pounds. It felt wonderful to get back to work and get off welfare, but my physical and emotional life was a mess. I desperately wanted to lose weight but was afraid of trying anything for fear it would just lead to gaining more.

"Then, I discovered the 3-Hour Diet™. Finally, I have found a program that makes sense! The food plan seemed easy for me to follow. I truly believed this program would work and that I was worth the effort. I realized I could no longer continue to live my life this way. I had had enough! I needed to change and I was willing to do whatever I had to. When I began the program, I lost 4 pounds the first week. I have now lost 70 pounds to date on the 3-Hour Diet™! Only 25 more pounds to my goal!

"I used to hate looking at myself in the mirror. I looked like an old, tired, fat woman and, I felt like an old, tired, fat woman. Now, I am truly amazed at my appearance. It still surprises me! I sometimes catch a glimpse of myself in a reflection and it takes me a minute to realize 'Hey, that's me!'"

Cathy's Secrets to Success

➤ Face your emotional issues head on rather than use food to solve them.
➤ Plan and prepare meals and snacks ahead of time.
➤ Get support from family and friends.
➤ Keep a scrap book that details your weight-loss journey.

extraordinary tasks every day, so you should give it the respect and love it deserves!

To love and respect your body, you must love yourself. You must become your own greatest friend. After all, who feeds you, puts you to sleep, and controls your life? You do. You are in control. Only when you ignite motivation to take care of yourself and treat yourself with the greatest care and respect will others be able to unconditionally support, nurture and comfort you.

To become your greatest friend, you must do three things:

• Accept your current self
• Ignite your deepest motivation
• Use a journal to express your feelings

Accept your current self

So many of my clients come to me and say they hate their bodies. Think about it: How do you treat something you hate? You ignore it, and that's what so many people who need to lose weight do. Instead of working to change the things they hate about their bodies, they focus their attention elsewhere.

And many people falsely think that as soon as they reach their goal weight, they'll start loving and respecting their bodies. This simply is not true. Some of the most tortured souls have the thinnest bodies. So if you think a smaller body will result in better body acceptance, you've put the cart before the horse because it's actually the reverse. As soon as you start loving and respecting your body, you'll have more success with becoming thin. In order to have a beautiful body, you must start to respect it *right now,* no matter how many pounds you currently need to lose.

Trust me on this: If you don't respect your body and treat it as the great

Is It Emotional or Is It Hunger?

Many of my 3-Hour Diet™ clients thought they were enslaved by emotional eating before they met me. They felt out of control at parties and when presented with treats. They found themselves raiding the fridge at night, and they simply couldn't get a handle on their eating.

As it turned out for many of them, however, the true problem wasn't necessarily emotional (although that certainly contributed to some of it). The true problem was hunger. Over the years, they had put themselves on one deprivation diet after another and had become very adept at starving themselves and punishing their bodies. They would eat very little all day long. Eventually their hunger would grow so great that they would give in—and stuff themselves with all of the foods they craved.

Simply switching to the 3-hour lifestyle solved these eating issues for many. Once they began nurturing their bodies by eating every 3 hours, they no longer felt ravenous at the end of the day, and found the willpower to walk away from cake, cookies, and other foods. "The biggest thing that has happened to me on the 3-Hour Diet™ is that I've forgotten about food," says one of my clients Celeste Roberts. Another client, Laura Porter says, "I thought I was an emotional eater. I thought I had psychological problems. It turned out that I just wasn't eating often enough. Now that I eat every 3 hours, I never eat emotionally."

So always remember to nurture yourself by eating every 3 hours. That's the first and most important strategy for eliminating emotional eating for good.

gift that it is, you will never find the willpower to do the things necessary to lose weight, such as stick to healthy food portions, drink plenty of water, and get enough sleep.

You must realize that you are good enough and amazing enough to lose weight—that you *deserve* to have a beautiful body. Once you do this, you will consistently make your health your #1 priority, you will effortlessly make the best decisions for your body, you will unlock deep and powerful feelings of motivation, and you'll learn the most important secret to shedding pounds and keeping them off forever!

Ignite your deepest motivation

Once you've learned to love and respect your current body, you will be ready to ignite your deepest motivation. To start, you must establish a specific goal.

You can never achieve success without having a specific goal or target to work toward. If you're looking for a new job, for instance, you must first identify the field in which you want to work and the areas where you want to live.

To set a goal for weight loss, you must first determine your happy weight. This will not only help you pinpoint a goal weight and a goal date by which to reach that weight; it will help you set mini-goals along the way, which will give you short-term goals to focus on.

If you have a lot of weight to lose, your goal date may seem far away, but you'll gain motivation by reaching your minigoals along the way. If you have 200 pounds to lose, at the safe rate of two pounds a week, it will take you 100 weeks. If you have 100 pounds to lose, it will take 50 weeks. For 30 pounds, it will take 15 weeks, and so on. But if you set achievable, shorter mini-goals, you'll have many reasons to celebrate your success as you move toward your goal weight! (See page 128.)

To keep your motivation high, I want you to reward yourself for each short- and long-term goal you reach. Make sure you pick a reward that has nothing to do with food, such as a manicure, pedicure, day at the spa, shopping spree, or vacation.

Another way to ignite your deepest motivation is to visualize yourself at your future goal weight. Take three photographs of yourself at your current weight in regular clothes—a front and a back or side shot—and paste them on page 128. These photos will act as a constant reminder of how much progress you've made toward your goal.

On a weight-loss journey, it's easy to feel discouraged and be tempted to slip back into old emotional eating habits. After all, you've conducted your life in a certain way for so long. Whenever you feel this way, look at your "before" photos. They don't lie!

And you may not have thought it possible, but thanks to an online tool, you can create "after" photographs of yourself as well! You don't actually have to lose the weight to see your future body—sort of a preview of what you're working so hard to achieve. Just go to www.myvirtualmodel.com and create a photograph of yourself at your future ideal weight. It's a revolutionary virtual photo technology created by a Canadian company called My Virtual Model Inc.

Print out the photographs of the future you from the front, side and back and paste them on the "after" spots on page 128. If you don't have on-line access, choose photographs of yourself before you gained weight or select images from magazines of models you'd like to resemble.

These "after" photographs will serve as a very powerful motivational force, perhaps more powerful than the "before" photographs. If you can visualize exactly what you're working toward, you will stay motivated and focused enough to achieve your goal.

It's also important that you get to know the future you. Visualize how your life will change once you reach your goal weight. Think about a typical day in the life of the future you. Starting from the moment you get out of bed, describe a day in the life of your future self. How do you feel when you get up? What do you wear? What do people say to you?

Although it may seem silly, this exercise will point you in the right direction and help motivate you to get to your future self. Just as motivational guru Stephen Covey has said, you have to begin with the end in mind. You must visualize your goal—in this case, a happier, slimmer, healthier you—before you start your journey toward achieving it.

Use a journal to express your feelings

It's one thing to experience a feeling; it's another to write it down. Putting your thoughts and feelings on paper validates them and makes them more concrete and real. Your notebook will listen without bias or judgment; it's like having a friend with you who loves and accepts you unconditionally at all times. Not to mention the therapeutic effects of expressing your thoughts this way; research shows that people who keep journals improve both their physical and emotional health. Writing down your feelings is one of the most important secrets to becoming your own greatest friend.

To start, designate a notebook as your weight-loss journal. Take this journal wherever you go and write in it every day. Describe every feeling you have, every challenge you face, and every temptation you have to go back to your old ways.

If you pass a fast food restaurant and have the urge to pull your car into the parking lot, pull over and express your desire for a cheeseburger in your notebook instead. If a bad day at the office sends your chocolate craving soaring, take your emotions to your notebook instead of the candy bar machine. Let your journal be your friend and turn to it whenever you feel depressed, sad, vulnerable, guilty, angry, or lonely.

Because I believe so strongly in the power of a weight-loss journal, I've included a space for you to write down your thoughts, feelings, successes, and failures in your planner in chapter 9.

A New Solution

If you're an emotional eater, you're most likely substituting cheeseburgers and chips for hugs and kisses. In other words, you eat because you're hungry for personal contact. In your times of need, if you had contacted a friend or loved one for a shoulder to cry on, you may not have cried over a bowl of ice cream.

Thing is, food doesn't ask you how you're feeling, give you hugs, or listen to you when you talk. To be frank, food doesn't care about you in the slightest. In order to get the kind of nurturing you really need—someone to say, "I love you and approve of who you are, no matter what"—you need people.

Studies have shown that contact with people is necessary from the moment we're born. Babies who have aloof and distant caregivers often develop what's called an *avoidant attachment style*, which causes them to have difficulty developing intimate relationships for the rest of their lives. And these babies can also suffer physically, and develop an immune deficiency known as "failure to thrive" syndrome that can lead to a severe handicap or even death.

Unfortunately, many of us are starved for human validation or acknowledgment, which is why so many of us are overweight. Many people who don't fill emotional voids with food turn to drugs or alcohol instead. If you are an emotional eater, you probably didn't get the nurturing you needed at some point in your life. Maybe your mom was too busy working to listen to you or spend time with you, or maybe your father left you when you were young.

No matter what the source of your emotional needs, you're never going to find it in a bowl or on a plate. You need people! As soon as you start filling your hungry heart with the comfort and support you crave—from people—you will no longer need to fill yourself up with food.

Luckily, I have a calorie-free, food-free method that will provide you with the kind of comfort and support you truly require. It's called the People Solution™. Now that you've examined the source of your emotional eating and started to accept yourself, you've started moving toward the People Solution.™

Build an Inner Support Team

For the People Solution™ to work, you must establish a support network of people to help you on your weight-loss journey. I call this network of peo-

RUTH WILSON—LOST 36 POUNDS

Height: 5'4"
Age: 53
Starting weight: 167 lbs.
Current weight: 131 lbs.
Other: A single mom with three kids

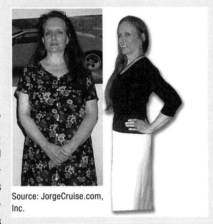

Source: JorgeCruise.com, Inc.

"When I was a child, I used to visit my grandparents' home with my parents. They spoke only Polish. There was nothing for a 5-year-old to do, so my sweet grandmother used to give me whole packages of cookies to eat in order to keep me occupied. Though she meant well, this is what I believe was the root of my lifetime of overeating.

"As time went by my habits grew worse. I tried different methods for weight loss, but none of them worked for me. I would lose some weight, only to gain it back.

"I decided to give Jorge's program a try. After a few weeks I joined his online club. It is so supportive! My wonderful son Adam has always cheered me on. He keeps telling me how proud he is of me with each step I make toward my goal.

"**I have gone from a size 12 to a size 6!** It's thrilling to feel so much healthier. I have learned many lessons, especially how to eat in moderation. This program is something I can live with, which is so important to my long-term success. I highly recommend it!"

Ruth's Secrets to Success

➤ Don't keep high-calorie temptations around, at least not in sight. Stock your kitchen with healthy foods.
➤ Get support from your family and look to them for inspiration. If you can't do it for yourself, do it for your kids.

ple your *inner support team*. This team can include family members, coworkers, and good friends—anyone who you feel comfortable communicating with openly and honestly. People in your inner support team must be caring and nonjudgmental. They must be willing to genuinely listen to you and support you.

Start by thinking of seven people you'd like to invite into your inner support team and list them in the space below.

MY SUPPORT TEAM

List the seven people on your support team in the spaces provided.

NAME	KIND	CONTACT INFO
1.		
2.		
3.		
4.		
5.		
6.		
7.		

Next you will place those seven people into the following buddy groups:

- 3 e-mail buddies
- 3 phone buddies
- 1 accountability buddy

If you can't think of seven people you would like to invite, just fill in as many as you can. Before you start contacting your buddies, you must first ask them to join your inner team. As an invitation, mail each buddy a very special "snail mail" letter asking for their help. Here's how each of the categories works:

E-mail buddies: Designate three of your seven people as e-mail buddies and fill their e-mail addresses in the contact information area. Anytime you feel the urge to eat in response to an emotion, e-mail your e-mail buddies and tell them about how you are feeling. For example, you might write, "I just had an argument with my teenage daughter because she came home late and I'm very upset. I feel like she has no respect for me, and all I want to do is raid the fridge." Ask your e-mail buddies to respond to your messages within twenty-four hours and offer comforting words.

Phone buddies: Designate another three of your seven people as phone buddies and fill in their home, work, and cell phone numbers in the contact information column. These buddies will help you put on the brakes when you need immediate support. The minute you feel yourself heading toward the kitchen, call the first buddy on your phone buddy list. He or she should know just what to say to strengthen your willpower and keep you from eating.

Accountability buddy: The last buddy on your inner support team is your accountability buddy. This person will help keep you accountable for your weight loss goal by talking to you for thirty minutes, once a week, preferably at the beginning of the week. Your accountability buddy should be someone whose lifestyle you admire—someone who is healthy and fit, someone to serve as a role model for you. Write your accountability buddy's contact information in the appropriate spot.

During your talks with your accountability buddy, you should discuss the number of pounds you've lost so far in total, the number of pounds you lost the previous week, and the two things you did that week that you're most proud of. For instance, maybe you took your niece or nephew to a carnival and bypassed every food tent with ease, or you successfully avoided eating after 7:30 every night.

Expand Your Inner Support Team

Now that you've built the shell of your inner support team with your phone buddies, e-mail buddies and accountability buddy, you can expand your support safety net by adding more people. After all, the more people you have to catch you, the safer you'll be if you fall.

To expand your inner support team, you can start your own weekly weight-loss group in your hometown or join my online weight loss club.

Create a Triad: You + 2 = Success

Many of my clients from both my books and my online weight loss club at JorgeCruise.com form what is called a *triad* to enhance their People Solution™. Three of my current clients, Karen, Michelle, and Annette, have supported each other through their weight-loss success and continue to keep each other accountable. You've already seen their individual success stories and "before" and "after" photos in earlier chapters.

Together they have already lost over 100 pounds, and are still losing. Many times a week, they meet online at JorgeCruise.com to chat and share their latest success. They have discovered that Them + 2 = success. This is a great way to focus on making the People Solution™ work for you. So get out there and form your triad.

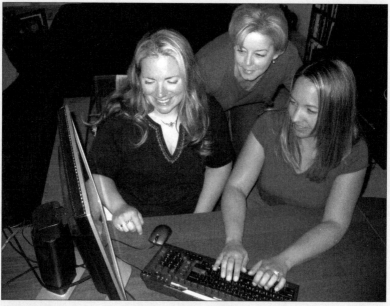

SOURCE: Jorge.Cruise.com

Creating a weight-loss group in your hometown will not only help you expand your inner support network, it will help you meet new people to socialize with as well.

A local bookstore is a great meeting place for your group. In fact, there are Jorge Cruise weight-loss groups already meeting in bookstores across the country.

If there isn't an established Jorge Cruise club near you, speak with the manager of a local bookstore, show him or her this book and explain that you'd like to start a weight-loss book club. I've received many e-mails from people who have started clubs and they're quite successful. And if I'm ever in your hometown, I might just have to stop by one of your meetings!

Stop the Sabotage Today

At this point, I'm sure you realize that you cannot successfully lose weight if you're feeding your hungry heart with food. The only way to stop emotional eating is to nourish your heart with the love and support it craves—the kind that comes from people.

To give your hungry heart a positive emotional jumpstart, commit five to ten minutes to nurturing and feeding it each morning. Review some of the supportive words in the e-mails from your e-mail buddies, or send a friend or loved one a quick message to let him or her know you're thinking about them.

And remember to show yourself some affection as well. Congratulate yourself for breaking out of the emotional eating trap. You will now enjoy true freedom long-term, no longer sabotage yourself, and break out of the food prison that once enslaved you!

Conquer the Night

Many of my clients tell me the most difficult time for them to conquer emotional eating comes after 7 P.M. They've eaten dinner, have few distractions, and have no one there to see them eat. They may be mentally stewing over something that happened earlier in the day, and they hear the fridge and the cupboards calling their name.

It generally starts innocently enough. They think they feel hungry and decide to eat something healthy, such as a hard-boiled egg or some sliced veggies. Invariably, that doesn't fill the void and they move on to something a little less healthy, perhaps some popcorn. That doesn't fill the void and before they know it they move on to the ice cream or cake.

The key to conquering this time of day is the same as any time of day: support. You must replace your craving for food with true comfort. You must remove the thorn that is driving you to eat. The only way to remove that thorn is to unload your feelings and face the true problem. If you often find yourself overeating at night, plan support into your evenings. Give yourself something to turn to instead of food. Try these strategies.

Join the JorgeCruise.com Online Club

In addition to your inner support network, you can find people to support you any time you log on your computer at JorgeCruise.com. Anytime you feel the urge to walk to the refrigerator, head over to your computer instead. There are numerous discussion boards and chat rooms on my Web site that allow you to link up with people all over the world.

My online club will also give you access to the following:

- Daily motivational messages
- Weekly online meetings
- Live chat auditoriums with myself and others
- Chat rooms for making new friends and supportive buddies
- Expert advice from others who have successfully lost weight on the 3-Hour Diet™

As soon as you finish dinner and your treat, go online. E-mail your weight-loss buddies, log on to weight-loss chat rooms, or e-mail friends and family members about your day. The key here is to unload the frustrations of the day, so that these frustrations no longer tempt you to enter the kitchen.

Write in your journal every evening. You may already feel called into the kitchen, but don't allow yourself to go there until after you've written in your journal. Write down the events of the day and how they made you feel. Write about your anger, sadness, hurts, and frustrations. Get it all out. Usually, by the time you are done, that loud voice from the kitchen will have diminished to a quiet whisper that will be much easier for you to ignore.

Call or meet a friend every evening. Find a trusted friend whom you can call each night to talk about your day. You can have these chats on the phone or have them during a walk around the neighborhood. The important thing is that you can open up fully, talking about your frustrations at work or even with your own family.

PART IV

Living the 3-Hour Lifestyle

28-DAY SUCCESS PLANNER

ntil recently, I avoided looking in the mirror. It made me ill when I saw how obese I'd become. Now, I'm the incredible shrinking woman! I check myself out in the mirror to see which parts are deflating this week! I'm trying on all the smaller-sized clothing in my closet that I haven't been able to wear for over 5 years! This has become a contest for my health. Following Jorge's 3-Hour Diet™ is a win-win situation for anyone that wants a real change in their health and body image. I started at a size 24, have lost 32 pounds (and counting!) and I can now fit in a size 16!!"

—LORI WIAR—LOST 32 POUNDS

Welcome to your 3-Hour Planner. What you will find in the next 126 pages will help you to stay motivated and organized for the next 28 days. I urge you to complete every task in your planner as indicated. They will all help you stay on track and achieve ultimate success.

Within your 28-day planner you will find the following:

- **A daily visualization.** A powerful mind/body technique, visualization helps you to create what you want in life. Too often, we use the power of visualization, somewhat unconsciously, in a negative way. We focus on negative concepts about life, which only work to fulfill that negative vision. In short, if you focus on the fat that you don't want, you'll end up with fat that you don't want!

  Keep in mind, the visualizations are meant to be beneficial for both men and women alike. Although some of the visualization in the 28-day planner are geared to women, the visualizations also will work for men. Men, all you have to do is use your imagination to visualize how they can be beneficial to you. For instance, on Day 1 visualize yourself as the best man in a wedding (not the maid of honor): You look so trim and handsome in that tuxedo and you know that everyone has noticed—how special that feels! Remember visualization is just that, and make it work for you.

  To truly visualize the new you, you must feel relaxed and calm. Your mind should be free of mental clutter to allow yourself to focus on your visualization. If you are not in a relaxed state, negative thoughts may pop up. Being relaxed allows the message to affect you more powerfully. So before each day's visualization, go to a quiet room in your house, play some soft music, and do whatever you need to do to relax.
- **A daily inspiring quote.** I hope these "Jorge-isms" will make you feel as if I am right there with you, coaching you in person.
- **A daily time-management tip.** For optimal success on the 3-Hour Diet™, you must use time wisely. These tips will help you create the time you need to prepare food and eat every 3 hours.
- **A daily eating 3-Hour Timeline™.** Ideally, you should write your meals into your planner at the beginning of every week. This will give you time to shop for the foods you need and to prepare various foods at the beginning of the week as needed. You can fill in your food planner by using the sample meals in chapter 13 or the 3-Hour Plate™. For snacks and treats, consult the food lists in chapter 12.
- **A weekly weigh-in reminder.** I encourage you to weigh yourself each Sunday and to write your weight in your planner. This will help you keep track of your success.

Your Homework

Before you get started on your new adventure, you'll need to make sure you have the tools for the journey. Please don't start the program until you have.

1. Written down your current weight and measurements and taken up to three "before" photos. Your original weight, waist circumference, and before photos will help serve not only as powerful reminders of your goal, but they will also help you to see your progress. To take your measurements, use a flexible tape measure. Wrap it around your waist, just above your hip bones. Record your answers in the space provided on "Your Current Body and Future Goals."

2. Determined your goal. Sure you want to lose weight, but how much? I recommend you pick a happy goal weight. That way you'll know when you've reached it! To pick a goal weight, consult the height and weight chart on page 129. Find your age on the chart and match that to your height. There you will find a healthy weight range for someone your age and size. Use that to determine your goal. Write your goal in the space provided on "Your Current Body and Future Goals." You also might want to choose a motivational goal as well, one that is not tied to the scale. For example, do you have a pair of jeans that you can no longer wear? You might want to write that down as a goal, too.

3. Determined how long it will take to reach your goal. You'll find out how to do just that by following the instructions in "Your Current Body and Future Goals."

4. Committed yourself to success. Too many people commit themselves half-heartedly to losing weight. They tell themselves, "Well, if this works out, great, but it's no big deal if it doesn't." They tell no one about their goal. That way, if they fail, no one will know it. If you don't make a firm commitment, you'll have a tough time sticking to the program. That's why I want you to fill out **"My Success Contract"** on page 130 right now. It will serve as a powerful reminder of your decision and will hold you accountable to the program.

Your Current Body and Future Goals

To find your goal weight, find your age and height on the chart on page 129. You know yourself better than anyone else does, so select a number that is realistic for you. Subtract that number from your current weight. That's your weight-loss goal.

Then, to determine a target date for achieving this goal, divide your weight-loss goal by 2. That's the number of weeks it will take to reach your goal. Consult a calendar and find the exact date you will achieve your *happy goal weight*.

Please record your answers to the following:

Current weight: _____

Current thigh circumference in inches: _____

Current hip circumference in inches: _____

Current waist circumference in inches: _____

Happy goal weight: _____

What date will you reach your goal weight: _____

Insert
"before"
photo
here

Insert
"before"
photo
here

YOUR HEALTHY WEIGHT

Use this chart and find a healthy weight range and choose your happy weight.

HEIGHT (FT/IN.) (AGE)	WEIGHT (LB)	
	19–34 YR	35+ YR
5'0"	97–128	108–138
5'1"	101–132	111–143
5'2"	104–137	115–148
5'3"	107–141	119–152
5'4"	111–146	122–157
5'5"	114–150	126–162
5'6"	118–155	130–167
5'7"	121–160	134–172
5'8"	125–164	138–178
5'9"	129–169	142–183
5'10"	132–174	146–188
5'11"	136–179	151–194
6'0"	140–184	155–199
6'1"	144–189	159–205
6'2"	148–195	164–210
6'3"	152–200	168–216

SOURCE: U.S. Department of Health and Human Services, Dietary Guidelines for Americans

NOTE: Some scales only go up to 280 pounds, so if you are over that in weight, it's difficult to get an accurate starting point. Here is my little secret I am sharing with you, straight from the mouths of my clients. If you need an extra-large weight capacity scale, Tanita® makes a great one. Go to www.tanita.com to find a store near you.

Don't forget to take your "before" photo! Who knows, you may be our next winner.

Here's what to do:

1) The day you begin the 3-Hour Diet, take your "before" pictures.

2) Lose the weight, get to your happy goal weight, and take some great "after" photos.

3) E-mail your story and all photos to stories@jorgecruise.com. Be sure to include your name, start weight, new weight, height, address, and phone number.

Each month we select one lucky success story submission to be flown to San Diego for an all-expense-paid *makeover* photo shoot. If you are selected, you will appear on the front page of JorgeCruise.com and/or in *First for Women* magazine or one of our future books, too. *So get ready to be a superstar!*

My 3-Hour Diet™ Success Contract

Filling out this contract will help keep you accountable to your goals. Make three copies and give them to three trusted friends who will support and motivate you in your journey to sucess.

Name: _____

Today's date: _____

I am going to weigh this many pounds: _____

By this date: _____

_____
Signature

Photocopy this contract and place on your refrigerator. Join JorgeCruise.com for support and to stay accountable.

"Don't say, 'If I could,
I would.' Say, 'If I can, I will.'"

—JIM ROHN, MOTIVATIONAL SPEAKER

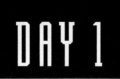

Today's Visualization

Today you are going to take a journey one year into the future. Close your eyes and take a few deep, relaxing breaths.

You are getting ready to attend a wedding for your best friend, and you are the maid or matron of honor or best man! See yourself pull the long, slinky dress out of your closet or admire your tuxedo. Drape your clothes over a chair and take a good look. How do you think you will look all dressed up for the special event? How do you think it will feel on your now-slimmer body?

Pull on your clothes and feel the fabric fall around your body. Notice how your dress or tuxedo feels, how no part of it bunches or grabs. It fits perfectly. Notice your slender arms and how shapely your shoulders are. Turn around and take in your rear view. How do you look? How do you feel?

Now, see yourself a few hours later, dancing at the wedding reception. Notice how all eyes are on you, admiring how you look. See a smile creep across your face. You've reached your goal and you look fantastic.

Your 3-Hour Plan

1) Commit your eating times.
2) Create your custom meals from the food lists starting on page 268 or from the premade meals starting on page 283.
3) Then keep your eye on this page and check off boxes when done eating.

☐ **Time:** | **Breakfast**

Veg/Fruit
Carbs
Protein   Fat

Custom Meal:
Carbs_____
Protein_____
Fat_____
Veg/Fruit_____

Premade Meal:_____

☐ **Time:** | **Snack A**

* If you weigh 200-249 lb. = double snack; 250-299 lb. = triple snack; 300+ = quadruple snack

☐ **Time:** | **Lunch**

Veg/Fruit
Carbs
Protein   Fat

Custom Meal:
Carbs_____
Protein_____
Fat_____
Veg/Fruit_____

Premade Meal:_____

☐ **Time:** | **Snack B**

* If you weigh 200-249 lb. = double snack; 250-299 lb. = triple snack; 300+ = quadruple snack

☐ **Time:** | **Dinner**

Veg/Fruit
Carbs
Protein   Fat

Custom Meal:
Carbs_____
Protein_____
Fat_____
Veg/Fruit_____

Premade Meal:_____

☐ **Time:** | **Treat**

Water

☐☐☐☐☐☐☐☐

Freebie Tracker

DAY 1

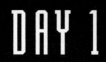

JORGE-ISM

"The 3-Hour Diet is practical so you won't sabotage yourself. You're going to get it this time! You're going to lose weight and keep it off. You are going to be successful."

3-Hour Timing Tip

*D*evelop a rotating menu system: To assist with meal planning and save time, plan out a whole month's worth of meals, snacks and treats and then just re-use the same plan each month. For example, you'll eat the same meals on August 15 as you did on July 15. You'll save hours trying to brainstorm new meal combinations.

Journal Notes

_____
_____
_____
_____
_____
_____
_____
_____
_____
_____
_____
_____
_____
_____
_____
_____
_____

"It's time to start living the
life you've imagined."

—HENRY JAMES, AUTHOR

Today's Visualization

Today you are going to see yourself at your goal weight, a few years in the future. Today is the day of your high school class reunion. You haven't seen most of your class-mates in many, many years. You are excited to show off what has become of you—how slim, healthy, and happy you are! It's time to get dressed. Imagine what you are wearing, what shoes you slip on your feet, what jewelry you put on, how you style your hair, what makeup you apply, and how you feel when you look in the mirror. You look great and feel fabulous!

As you approach the entrance of the reunion, take a deep breath and then confidently glide into the room. Whom do you see from high school and what do they say to you? Hear the compliments and "oohs" and "ahs." Tell your classmates how terrific you feel. Later in the evening, a class picture is taken. See yourself, standing tall, lean, and confident amongst your high school classmates.

Your 3-Hour Plan

1) Commit your eating times.
2) Create your custom meals from the food lists starting on page 268 or from the premade meals starting on page 283.
3) Then keep your eye on this page and check off boxes when done eating.

☐ **Time:** ▮ **Breakfast**

Custom Meal:
Carbs_____
Protein_____
Fat_____
Veg/Fruit_____

Premade Meal:_____

☐ **Time:** ▮ **Snack A**

* If you weigh 200-249 lb. = double snack; 250-299 lb. = triple snack; 300+ = quadruple snack

☐ **Time:** ▮ **Lunch**

Custom Meal:
Carbs_____
Protein_____
Fat_____
Veg/Fruit_____

Premade Meal:_____

☐ **Time:** ▮ **Snack B**

* If you weigh 200-249 lb. = double snack; 250-299 lb. = triple snack; 300+ = quadruple snack

☐ **Time:** ▮ **Dinner**

Custom Meal:
Carbs_____
Protein_____
Fat_____
Veg/Fruit_____

Premade Meal:_____

☐ **Time:** ▮ **Treat**

Water

Freebie Tracker

DAY 2

3-Hour Timing Tip

Make a master shopping list: If you have a regular monthly menu, you can also reuse grocery lists. If you do your grocery shopping once a week, plan out four permanent shopping lists, photocopy them, and reuse them. If you do your shopping every two weeks, you'll only have to create two permanent lists.

Journal Notes

_____

_____

_____

_____

_____

_____

_____

_____

_____

_____

_____

_____

_____

_____

_____

_____

_____

_____

"We all have the extraordinary coded inside us, waiting to be released."

—JEAN HOUSTON, PSYCHOANALYST

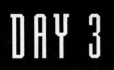

DAY 3

Today's Visualization

I t's time to get dressed up in your finest attire because tonight you are going to shine at a very elegant, formal affair! You are going to wear that little black dress, the one you've kept in the back of your closet for when you had a body to show off. So, close your eyes and take a few relaxing breaths, in through your nose and out through your mouth.

See yourself getting ready for your special occasion. See the black dress hanging in your closet. Walk over to it. Take it out of the closet and drape it over the front of your body. Feel yourself growing excited at the prospect of finally wearing the dress. Lay the dress on your bed and notice every detail about it. Think back to the last time you wore it. How long ago was that? Then pick it up and slip it on. Feel the silky material fall evenly over your body. Put on your shoes and take a look at yourself in the mirror. See your belly, how nothing bulges. See your slender, toned arms. Then, fast forward to your big event. See yourself in the ballroom. Sense all of the eyes on you. You are confident and stunning. Dance the night away and enjoy it!

Your 3-Hour Plan

1) Commit your eating times.
2) Create your custom meals from the food lists starting on page 268 or from the premade meals starting on page 283.
3) Then keep your eye on this page and check off boxes when done eating.

☐ Time: **Breakfast**

Veg/Fruit
Carbs
Protein   Fat

Custom Meal:
Carbs_____
Protein_____
Fat_____
Veg/Fruit_____

Premade Meal:_____

☐ Time: **Snack A**

* If you weigh 200-249 lb. = double snack; 250-299 lb. = triple snack; 300+ = quadruple snack

☐ Time: **Lunch**

Veg/Fruit
Carbs
Protein   Fat

Custom Meal:
Carbs_____
Protein_____
Fat_____
Veg/Fruit_____

Premade Meal:_____

☐ Time: **Snack B**

* If you weigh 200-249 lb. = double snack; 250-299 lb. = triple snack; 300+ = quadruple snack

☐ Time: **Dinner**

Veg/Fruit
Carbs
Protein   Fat

Custom Meal:
Carbs_____
Protein_____
Fat_____
Veg/Fruit_____

Premade Meal:_____

☐ Time: **Treat**

Water

Freebie Tracker

DAY 3

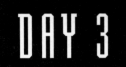
JORGE-ISM

"Many people are too hard on themselves when trying to lose weight. Be patient. The weight will come off. It might not come off overnight, but it will come off."

3-Hour Timing Tip

*T*ry to keep breakfast simple: There are many quick, healthful breakfast foods available, so you can save time and energy by keeping this meal relatively simple. Stick with things like high-fiber cereal, whole-grain toast, oatmeal, and fruit—things you can throw together in just a few minutes. Then concentrate harder on your lunches and dinners.

Journal Notes

_____

_____

_____

_____

_____

_____

_____

_____

_____

_____

_____

_____

_____

_____

_____

_____

_____

_____

"If you hear a voice within you say 'you cannot paint,' by all means paint, and that voice will be silenced."

—VINCENT VAN GOGH, ARTIST

Today's Visualization

Today is a glorious summer day filled with sunshine and warm breezes. It's the perfect day to hit the beach with a few of your friends during a very relaxing visualization exercise. Close your eyes and take a few relaxing breaths, in through your nose and out through your mouth.

You've just gotten off the phone with your friend and you've decided to go spend the day at the beach. You haven't been to the beach in many years, ever since you became too embarrassed to wear a swimsuit in public. But now you've got a beautiful body. So slip on your swimsuit, flip-flops, and wide-brimmed straw hat. You and your friend sing along to oldies music on the way to the beach. Once there, you sink your toes into the hot sand and let out a deep sigh of delight. Doesn't it feel great? As you bare down to your bathing suit and spread out on your towel, you feel confident and beautiful. Feel the warm rays on your back and give your buddy a wink. She comments on how great you look and you reply with a heartfelt "thank you" and tell her just how great you feel. The two of you spend the afternoon gossiping on your beach towel, frolicking in the waves and strolling the length of the water's edge.

Your 3-Hour Plan

1) Commit your eating times.
2) Create your custom meals from the food lists starting on page 268 or from the premade meals starting on page 283.
3) Then keep your eye on this page and check off boxes when done eating.

☐ **Time:** _____ | **Breakfast**

Veg/Fruit
Carbs
Protein | Fat

Custom Meal:
Carbs_____
Protein_____
Fat_____
Veg/Fruit_____

Premade Meal:_____

☐ **Time:** _____ | **Snack A**

* If you weigh 200-249 lb. = double snack; 250-299 lb. = triple snack; 300+ = quadruple snack

☐ **Time:** _____ | **Lunch**

Veg/Fruit
Carbs
Protein | Fat

Custom Meal:
Carbs_____
Protein_____
Fat_____
Veg/Fruit_____

Premade Meal:_____

☐ **Time:** _____ | **Snack B**

* If you weigh 200-249 lb. = double snack; 250-299 lb. = triple snack; 300+ = quadruple snack

☐ **Time:** _____ | **Dinner**

Veg/Fruit
Carbs
Protein | Fat

Custom Meal:
Carbs_____
Protein_____
Fat_____
Veg/Fruit_____

Premade Meal:_____

☐ **Time:** _____ | **Treat**

Water

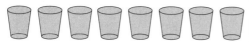

Freebie Tracker

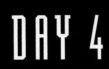

DAY 4

JORGE-ISM

"Once you get used to eating every three hours, your stomach will tell you when to eat. Our body sends us natural cues all of the time. We just need to tune in and listen."

3-Hour Timing Tip

Cook food ahead of time: Do as much food preparation as you can on the weekends, and then just freeze foods for later use. You'll save time by preparing food when everything is already spread out in front of you instead of taking everything out and putting it away seven days a week.

Journal Notes

_____

_____

_____

_____

_____

_____

_____

_____

_____

_____

_____

_____

_____

_____

_____

_____

_____

_____

_____

"Everyone has in them
something precious that
is in no one else."

—MARTIN BUBER, PHILOSOPHER

DAY 5

Today's Visualization

Close your eyes and take a few relaxing breaths—in through your nose and out through your mouth. Smile and jump into the future with me.

I want you to visualize yourself after you've reached your goal. Notice your entire body. See how fit and firm your arms have become. Notice your vibrant skin. Visualize how your clothes will fall on your body and how your shoes will fit. Imagine the colors, the textures, and the patterns of a favorite outfit that you will be wearing. What does the new you look like? Will you have a new haircut, new look, or new accessories? See your body doing different movements. See yourself walking, sitting at work, or driving in your car. Try to visualize every detail. You've got to smell, hear, touch, and taste your vision to make it a reality.

Your 3-Hour Plan

1) Commit your eating times.
2) Create your custom meals from the food lists starting on page 268 or from the premade meals starting on page 283.
3) Then keep your eye on this page and check off boxes when done eating.

☐ **Time:** _____ **Breakfast**

Veg/Fruit
Carbs
Protein   Fat

Custom Meal:
Carbs _____
Protein _____
Fat _____
Veg/Fruit _____

Premade Meal: _____

☐ **Time:** _____ **Snack A**

* If you weigh 200-249 lb. = double snack; 250-299 lb. = triple snack; 300+ = quadruple snack

☐ **Time:** _____ **Lunch**

Veg/Fruit
Carbs
Protein   Fat

Custom Meal:
Carbs _____
Protein _____
Fat _____
Veg/Fruit _____

Premade Meal: _____

☐ **Time:** _____ **Snack B**

* If you weigh 200-249 lb. = double snack; 250-299 lb. = triple snack; 300+ = quadruple snack

☐ **Time:** _____ **Dinner**

Veg/Fruit
Carbs
Protein   Fat

Custom Meal:
Carbs _____
Protein _____
Fat _____
Veg/Fruit _____

Premade Meal: _____

☐ **Time:** _____ **Treat**

Water

☐ ☐ ☐ ☐ ☐ ☐ ☐ ☐

Freebie Tracker

DAY 5

JORGE-ISM

"Sometimes we're embarrassed to tell others that we need support. Most people, however, are very helpful once they understand why you are trying this new way of eating, and they will help you get to your goal."

3-Hour Timing Tip

C lean out your kitchen: You can't be your most productive in your kitchen if it's filled with clutter and old appliances. So give your kitchen a mini-makeover. Donate appliances you have duplicates of, like blenders and electric mixers. And if you can afford it, replace old, antiquated appliances with newer, sleeker ones.

Journal Notes

_____

_____

_____

_____

_____

_____

_____

_____

_____

_____

_____

_____

_____

_____

_____

_____

_____

"Kites rise highest against
the wind—not with it."

—SIR WINSTON CHURCHILL

DAY 6

Today's Visualization

Close your eyes and take a few relaxing breaths—in through your nose and out through your mouth. Smile and jump into the future with me. Visualize the day that you reach your goal.

See yourself jump out of bed. As you get dressed, notice how you look. See your new sexy arms, legs, and torso. Go ahead and get dressed, making sure to pick that outfit you've always wanted to wear, but couldn't because of your weight. Notice how your clothes drape loosely over your body. Feel how none of the fabric hugs you or feels tight. Touch your body with your hands. How does it feel? Walk around. Notice that your thighs no longer rub together.

Look in the mirror and see how extraordinary you look and feel. What quality about your new self are you most proud of?

Smile. You've reached your goal!

Your 3-Hour Plan

1) Commit your eating times.
2) Create your custom meals from the food lists starting on page 268 or from the premade meals starting on page 283.
3) Then keep your eye on this page and check off boxes when done eating.

☐ **Time:** _____ | **Breakfast**

Veg/Fruit
Carbs
Protein   Fat

Custom Meal:
Carbs_____
Protein_____
Fat_____
Veg/Fruit_____

Premade Meal:_____

☐ **Time:** _____ | **Snack A**

---

* If you weigh 200-249 lb. = double snack; 250-299 lb. = triple snack; 300+ = quadruple snack

☐ **Time:** _____ | **Lunch**

Veg/Fruit
Carbs
Protein   Fat

Custom Meal:
Carbs_____
Protein_____
Fat_____
Veg/Fruit_____

Premade Meal:_____

☐ **Time:** _____ | **Snack B**

---

* If you weigh 200-249 lb. = double snack; 250-299 lb. = triple snack; 300+ = quadruple snack

☐ **Time:** _____ | **Dinner**

Veg/Fruit
Carbs
Protein   Fat

Custom Meal:
Carbs_____
Protein_____
Fat_____
Veg/Fruit_____

Premade Meal:_____

☐ **Time:** _____ | **Treat**

Water

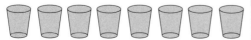

Freebie Tracker

DAY 6

3-Hour Timing Tip

Streamline your food prep: Preparing and packing your meals ahead of time requires a lot of slicing, dicing, and chopping. So think about investing in some appliances that will save you the time of doing all this, like a food processor, blender, garlic press, apple slicer, and so on.

Journal Notes

_____

_____

_____

_____

_____

_____

_____

_____

_____

_____

_____

_____

_____

_____

_____

_____

_____

_____

"You are the one who can
stretch your own horizon."

—EDGAR MAGNIN, RABBI

DAY 7

Today's Visualization

Today we will nurture your inner motivation with a very special visualization exercise. During today's visualization, you will be reunited with an old friend who hasn't seen you for many years. So, close your eyes and take a few relaxing breaths, in through your nose and out through your mouth.

See yourself pulling into the parking garage at the airport to pick up your friend. Take a quick look in the rear view and smile at your reflection. You look healthier, happier, and younger than you have in years! As you wait for the elevator, take a peek at your watch. You only have a few minutes until your friend's flight is due at the gate. You quickly head to the stairs and mount them two at a time. Feel how agile and strong your body feels as you quickly climb each staircase. Doesn't it feel wonderful to be able to move quickly without feeling out of breath? You make it to the gate just in time to see your friend approach. She smiles politely, says "Excuse me," and brushes past you. She doesn't recognize you! You call her name and say, "It's me!" Your friend turns around stunned and says, "You look incredible! What have you done?" You smile radiantly.

Your 3-Hour Plan

1) Commit your eating times.
2) Create your custom meals from the food lists starting on page 268 or from the premade meals starting on page 283.
3) Then keep your eye on this page and check off boxes when done eating.

☐ **Time:** _____ **Breakfast**

Veg/Fruit
Carbs
Protein   Fat

Custom Meal:
Carbs_____
Protein_____
Fat_____
Veg/Fruit_____
Premade Meal:_____

☐ **Time:** _____ **Snack A**

* If you weigh 200-249 lb. = double snack; 250-299 lb. = triple snack; 300+ = quadruple snack

☐ **Time:** _____ **Lunch**

Veg/Fruit
Carbs
Protein   Fat

Custom Meal:
Carbs_____
Protein_____
Fat_____
Veg/Fruit_____
Premade Meal:_____

☐ **Time:** _____ **Snack B**

* If you weigh 200-249 lb. = double snack; 250-299 lb. = triple snack; 300+ = quadruple snack

☐ **Time:** _____ **Dinner**

Veg/Fruit
Carbs
Protein   Fat

Custom Meal:
Carbs_____
Protein_____
Fat_____
Veg/Fruit_____
Premade Meal:_____

☐ **Time:** _____ **Treat**

Water

Freebie Tracker

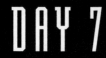

DAY 7

JORGE-ISM

"If you slip up, just get back on the program. You haven't lost the battle until you've quit."

3-Hour Timing Tip

*D*elegate household tasks: The more household chores you delegate to your family members, the more time you'll save. So don't be afraid to ask your son to clean the bathrooms once a week or your husband to dust the furniture. And once you delegate a task, let it go. Don't try to do it over or do it better, or you'll inherit the chore once again.

Journal Notes

_____

_____

_____

_____

_____

_____

_____

_____

_____

_____

_____

_____

_____

_____

_____

_____

_____

_____

_____

_____

_____

_____

_____

_____

_____

_____

_____

_____

_____

_____

_____

_____

_____

_____

_____

NOTE: Join JorgeCruise.com to track your meals online and for community support.

Weigh In

My current weight is:

Age: 38
Starting Weight: 245 lbs.
Current Weight: 195 lbs.
Other: A father of 3 small children; works
   as an interpreter and actor

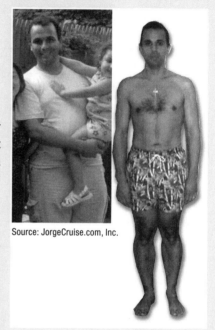

Source: JorgeCruise.com, Inc.

"Before the 3-Hour Diet™, I was no longer comfortable with my body. At first I thought it was part of getting older and being a dad. My acting career was at a standstill. I was a dad who had no energy for his kids. I decided to start working on myself.

"First I looked for an acting audition coach. Once I found her, I worked on my craft and got my acting confidence up. I worked with her for a few months and booked a small role on a primetime show (*Law & Order: SVU*). I was playing a morgue assistant and when they asked me what size scrubs they thought I wore, I told them large. I was wrong. They had to get me an XL. I was not happy. When I saw my brief moment on television I saw a fuller face than I was expecting.

"I started the 3-Hour Diet™ as a birthday gift to myself and have now been doing Jorge's program consistently for a year.

"My routine starts at six in the morning. I do my 8 Minutes Moves®, and about three or four days a week I go to the gym for 20 minutes to do the elliptical machine. Becoming a father for the third time has really tested my resolve. I have had a little sleep deprivation, but certainly not as bad as my wife. Over the weeks all of us have adjusted well.

"I have now become a sort of poster child for Jorge's program in my neighborhood, at my job, and to family members. **I feel motivated because I have motivated others.**"

Dennis's Secrets to Success

- ➤ If you have kids, aim to set a good example for them.
- ➤ Watch television programs that make you think about your health, such as those offered on Discovery Health.
- ➤ Make your morning exercises a routine, as routine as brushing your teeth. If you can, do the exercises right in the bathroom after you brush your teeth.

"Give your dreams all you've got and you'll be amazed at the energy that comes out of you."

—WILLIAM JAMES, PSYCHOLOGIST

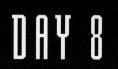

DAY 8

Today's Visualization

Today you will strengthen your motivation by visualizing your self in the future, after you have reached your goal. Today, you're preparing for a very special date. So, first relax by closing your eyes and taking a few deep, relaxing breaths, in through your nose and out through your mouth.

See yourself getting ready for your date. Who will be your date for the evening? How do you prepare for your date? See yourself taking a hot bubble bath with a glass of champagne or splurging on a manicure and facial or a long hot shower. Then, see yourself pick out your outfit. Find something special in the back of your closet, an outfit that you've always loved but one that you refused to wear because of your body. Maybe it has a slit high up on the leg or is a form-fitting dress shirt. Put it on. See how great your legs look in this outfit! Notice how the fabric touches against your toned skin. Look in the mirror and twirl around and smile at how slim and healthy you look.

Hear doorbell ring. Open the door and see your date. Hear your date comment about how lovely you look. What does your date say and how does it make you feel?

Your 3-Hour Plan

1) Commit your eating times.
2) Create your custom meals from the food lists starting on page 268 or from the premade meals starting on page 283.
3) Then keep your eye on this page and check off boxes when done eating.

☐ **Time:** _____ **Breakfast**

Veg/Fruit
Carbs
Protein Fat

Custom Meal:
Carbs_____
Protein_____
Fat_____
Veg/Fruit_____

Premade Meal:_____

☐ **Time:** _____ **Snack A**

* If you weigh 200-249 lb. = double snack; 250-299 lb. = triple snack; 300+ = quadruple snack

☐ **Time:** _____ **Lunch**

Veg/Fruit
Carbs
Protein Fat

Custom Meal:
Carbs_____
Protein_____
Fat_____
Veg/Fruit_____

Premade Meal:_____

☐ **Time:** _____ **Snack B**

* If you weigh 200-249 lb. = double snack; 250-299 lb. = triple snack; 300+ = quadruple snack

☐ **Time:** _____ **Dinner**

Veg/Fruit
Carbs
Protein Fat

Custom Meal:
Carbs_____
Protein_____
Fat_____
Veg/Fruit_____

Premade Meal:_____

☐ **Time:** _____ **Treat**

_____

Water

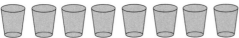

Freebie Tracker

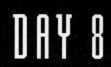

DAY 8

3-Hour Timing Tip

*A*void postponing important tasks: Don't put off things that you're not looking forward to doing. They will only come back to haunt you. Things rarely are more fun when you postpone them. Allow plenty of time for big, important jobs and make them less daunting by breaking them down into smaller tasks over time.

Journal Notes

_____

_____

_____

_____

_____

_____

_____

_____

_____

_____

_____

_____

_____

_____

_____

_____

"Motivation is what gets you started. Habit is what keeps you going."

—UNKNOWN

DAY 9

Today's Visualization

It's such a beautiful summer day out, so today you will accompany a friend and her dog to the park for a day of sunshine and playing around. Get ready by closing your eyes and taking a few deep, relaxing breaths, in through your nose and out through your mouth.

See yourself rubbing sunscreen onto your lean legs, firm arms, and smooth face. Being active is a way of life for you. Feel the enjoyment from deep inside that comes from spending the day outdoors being active. You straighten your visor, grab a water bottle from the fridge, and step out your front door just as your friend, and her pup, Kobe, are crossing the street. You jog down your front steps to greet them and give your friend a big hug.

The three of you walk the mile or so to the park, talking and laughing the whole way. As you enter the park, you stop off at a water fountain to refill your bottle and take a nice, long, refreshing sip. "Ahhhhh, that hits the spot!" you say. You head toward a big open lawn. Your buddy and you throw a Frisbee® and chase Kobe around the park. How great does it feel to be able to run and jump and play like a kid again?

Your 3-Hour Plan

1) Commit your eating times.
2) Create your custom meals from the food lists starting on page 268 or from the premade meals starting on page 283.
3) Then keep your eye on this page and check off boxes when done eating.

☐ Time: _____ | **Breakfast**

Veg/Fruit
Carbs
Protein   Fat

Custom Meal:
Carbs_____
Protein_____
Fat_____
Veg/Fruit_____

Premade Meal:_____

☐ Time: _____ | **Snack A**

_____
* If you weigh 200-249 lb. = double snack; 250-299 lb. = triple snack; 300+ = quadruple snack

☐ Time: _____ | **Lunch**

Veg/Fruit
Carbs
Protein   Fat

Custom Meal:
Carbs_____
Protein_____
Fat_____
Veg/Fruit_____

Premade Meal:_____

☐ Time: _____ | **Snack B**

_____
* If you weigh 200-249 lb. = double snack; 250-299 lb. = triple snack; 300+ = quadruple snack

☐ Time: _____ | **Dinner**

Veg/Fruit
Carbs
Protein   Fat

Custom Meal:
Carbs_____
Protein_____
Fat_____
Veg/Fruit_____

Premade Meal:_____

☐ Time: _____ | **Treat**

_____

Water

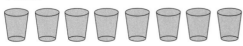

Freebie Tracker

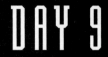

DAY 9

3-Hour Timing Tip

Keep a running list of projects you want to get to: If you continuously keep on top of the long-term big and small tasks you want to get to, you can use the time in between more immediate tasks to get them done. For example, maybe you've been meaning to organize your photos into albums.

When you have some time in between your day-to-day duties, you can start to fill it in by tackling the photos.

Journal Notes

_____

_____

_____

_____

_____

_____

_____

_____

_____

_____

_____

_____

_____

_____

_____

_____

_____

_____

"The best way to predict your future is to create it."

—UNKNOWN

DAY 10

Today's Visualization

For today's visualization exercise, you're going to feel the breeze run through your hair as you and a friend take a leisurely bike ride through your neighborhood. Get ready to hop on for a fun-filled ride! Close your eyes and take a few relaxing breaths, in through your nose and out through your mouth.

Picture yourself dressed in a pair of comfortable spandex shorts and a nice, cool cotton T-shirt. You're doing a few stretches as you wait for your friend to arrive at your house. See yourself in a sky-reaching pose: standing tall with both hands reaching up towards the blue sky. Feel the stretch lengthening your spine as you take a deep breath. See your friend steer her bike into the driveway.

You wheel your bike around the side of your house and think about how fun it is to be able to enjoy a day of bike riding. See yourself buckle the strap of your helmet under your chin, secure your water bottle into its holder, and pedal your bike out of your driveway. You and your friend pedal along, talking and laughing. Sometimes you ride slowly and leisurely, and other times you pick up the pace and playfully race one another. You feel like a kid again as you glide through your neighborhood, enjoying the scenery and the sun on your face.

Your 3-Hour Plan

1) Commit your eating times.
2) Create your custom meals from the food lists starting on page 268 or from the premade meals starting on page 283.
3) Then keep your eye on this page and check off boxes when done eating.

☐ Time: _____ **Breakfast**

Veg/Fruit
Carbs
Protein   Fat

Custom Meal:
Carbs_____
Protein_____
Fat_____
Veg/Fruit_____

Premade Meal:_____

☐ Time: _____ **Snack A**

---

* If you weigh 200-249 lb. = double snack; 250-299 lb. = triple snack; 300+ = quadruple snack

☐ Time: _____ **Lunch**

Veg/Fruit
Carbs
Protein   Fat

Custom Meal:
Carbs_____
Protein_____
Fat_____
Veg/Fruit_____

Premade Meal:_____

☐ Time: _____ **Snack B**

---

* If you weigh 200-249 lb. = double snack; 250-299 lb. = triple snack; 300+ = quadruple snack

☐ Time: _____ **Dinner**

Veg/Fruit
Carbs
Protein   Fat

Custom Meal:
Carbs_____
Protein_____
Fat_____
Veg/Fruit_____

Premade Meal:_____

☐ Time: _____ **Treat**

Water

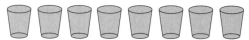

Freebie Tracker

DAY 10

3-Hour Timing Tip

*A*void interruptions: If you just can't stop playing computer games when you sit in front of your PC, step away from it. If you just have to get some food preparation and planning done for your 3-Hour Diet™ and your cell phone keeps ringing, turn it off. The best way to dodge interruptions is to avoid them in the first place.

Journal Notes

_____

_____

_____

_____

_____

_____

_____

_____

_____

_____

_____

_____

_____

_____

_____

_____

_____

_____

"Picture in your mind a sense
of personal destiny."

—WAYNE OATES, THEOLOGIAN AND PASTOR

3

Today's Visualization

Visualize yourself one year in the future. Close your eyes and take a few relaxing breaths, in through your nose and out through your mouth. See yourself as you would like to be. You are accomplishing all of the things that you'd like to accomplish in life with strength and vigor. You are focusing on what's most important to you, learning what you'd like to learn, and making your mark on the world.

What does this new world look like? What new mental, physical, and spiritual qualities have you uncovered? What lessons have you learned? What accomplishments are you most proud of? What did you develop inside of yourself to be able to accomplish so much? What was most important in helping you achieve your success? What helped you overcome any challenges along the way?

With those answers, take a step back to the present moment and visualize what you must do right now to make your future passions become a reality.

Your 3-Hour Plan

1) Commit your eating times.
2) Create your custom meals from the food lists starting on page 268 or from the premade meals starting on page 283.
3) Then keep your eye on this page and check off boxes when done eating.

☐ **Time:** _____ | **Breakfast**

Veg/Fruit
Carbs
Protein Fat

Custom Meal:
Carbs_____
Protein_____
Fat_____
Veg/Fruit_____

Premade Meal:_____

☐ **Time:** _____ | **Snack A**

_____
* If you weigh 200-249 lb. = double snack; 250-299 lb. = triple snack; 300+ = quadruple snack

☐ **Time:** _____ | **Lunch**

Veg/Fruit
Carbs
Protein Fat

Custom Meal:
Carbs_____
Protein_____
Fat_____
Veg/Fruit_____

Premade Meal:_____

☐ **Time:** _____ | **Snack B**

_____
* If you weigh 200-249 lb. = double snack; 250-299 lb. = triple snack; 300+ = quadruple snack

☐ **Time:** _____ | **Dinner**

Veg/Fruit
Carbs
Protein Fat

Custom Meal:
Carbs_____
Protein_____
Fat_____
Veg/Fruit_____

Premade Meal:_____

☐ **Time:** _____ | **Treat**

_____

Water

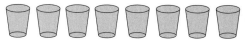

Freebie Tracker

DAY 11

JORGE-ISM

"Consider these statistics: The same percentage of Americans who are overweight—65 percent— also have no routine. If you can start and keep a routine, you will achieve success."

3-Hour Timing Tip

*D*on't be afraid to say "no": Whether it's to a social event or an extracurricular activity, saying no is not a crime. There is no harm in turning down invitations or simply saying, "I'm sorry, I can't" in order to get food shopping or other necessary chores finished. If you plan appropriately, you'll have time for the parties and events you *really* want to go to.

Journal Notes

_____

_____

_____

_____

_____

_____

_____

_____

_____

_____

_____

_____

_____

_____

_____

"You've got to get up every morning with determination if you're going to go to bed with satisfaction."

—GEORGE HORACE LORIMER, EDITOR

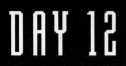

Today's Visualization

Close your eyes and take a few relaxing breaths, in through your nose and out through your mouth. Imagine you will soon be introduced to a buddy of your close friend for the first time. Let's say his name is Joe. Your friend and Joe have gotten together for coffee one day and your name has come up. Your friend says to Joe, "Oh yes, you have to meet her. She is a great friend and just a wonderful person." Joe asks, "How come? What makes her so great?" Visualize what your friend says next. What does your friend say about you? Does she talk about how you are always there with a hug or a smile when she needs you? Or does she tell a funny story about a time when you two had a ball together? Does she say that you are understanding and compassionate? Or steadfast and coura-geous? Or maybe that you have a great sense of humor or quick wit? When Joe asks what you look like, hear how your friend describes you, from your hair color to your toned legs, from your beauty mark to your great eyes. Smile, because you know your friend loves you very much.

Your 3-Hour Plan

1) Commit your eating times.
2) Create your custom meals from the food lists starting on page 268 or from the premade meals starting on page 283.
3) Then keep your eye on this page and check off boxes when done eating.

☐ **Time:** _____ **Breakfast**

Veg/Fruit
Carbs
Protein   Fat

Custom Meal:
Carbs_____
Protein_____
Fat_____
Veg/Fruit_____

Premade Meal:_____

☐ **Time:** _____ **Snack A**

---
* If you weigh 200-249 lb. = double snack; 250-299 lb. = triple snack; 300+ = quadruple snack
---

☐ **Time:** _____ **Lunch**

Veg/Fruit
Carbs
Protein   Fat

Custom Meal:
Carbs_____
Protein_____
Fat_____
Veg/Fruit_____

Premade Meal:_____

☐ **Time:** _____ **Snack B**

---
* If you weigh 200-249 lb. = double snack; 250-299 lb. = triple snack; 300+ = quadruple snack
---

☐ **Time:** _____ **Dinner**

Veg/Fruit
Carbs
Protein   Fat

Custom Meal:
Carbs_____
Protein_____
Fat_____
Veg/Fruit_____

Premade Meal:_____

☐ **Time:** _____ **Treat**

Water

Freebie Tracker

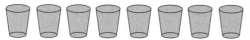

DAY 12

3-Hour Timing Tip

Put things in good places: When deciding where to put something, ask yourself, "Where would I look for this?" instead of "Where should I put this?" If you think about a good spot for something ahead of time, you'll save the time spent looking under beds and tearing apart closets to search for them later.

Journal Notes

_____

_____

_____

_____

_____

_____

_____

_____

_____

_____

_____

_____

_____

"Believe that you have it,
and you have it."

—LATIN PROVERB

DAY 13

Today's Visualization

Today you are getting ready for a Halloween party, and you must wear a disguise. What will you wear? Close your eyes and take a few relaxing breaths, in through your nose and out through your mouth. See all of your old frumpy Halloween outfits in your closet. Pull them out and put them in a pile for the Goodwill. You need an outfit that shows off the new you! Take yourself to the costume store. It's time to go shopping!

Find a sleek, sexy Halloween outfit at the store and try it on. Perhaps you chose the catwoman outfit or the Hooters® girl get-up. Regardless, try it on and see how it shows off all of your good qualities. Notice how, for the first time in years, you are not embarrassed to show off your body.

Take off the outfit and walk to the register to purchase it. See yourself smile. You look fantastic!

Your 3-Hour Plan

1) Commit your eating times.
2) Create your custom meals from the food lists starting on page 268 or from the premade meals starting on page 283.
3) Then keep your eye on this page and check off boxes when done eating.

| ☐ Time: | Breakfast |

Custom Meal:
Carbs_____
Protein_____
Fat_____
Veg/Fruit_____

Premade Meal:_____

| ☐ Time: | Snack A |

* If you weigh 200-249 lb. = double snack; 250-299 lb. = triple snack; 300+ = quadruple snack

| ☐ Time: | Lunch |

Custom Meal:
Carbs_____
Protein_____
Fat_____
Veg/Fruit_____

Premade Meal:_____

| ☐ Time: | Snack B |

* If you weigh 200-249 lb. = double snack; 250-299 lb. = triple snack; 300+ = quadruple snack

| ☐ Time: | Dinner |

Custom Meal:
Carbs_____
Protein_____
Fat_____
Veg/Fruit_____

Premade Meal:_____

| ☐ Time: | Treat |

Water

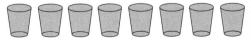

Freebie Tracker

DAY 13

"If you say 'I will,' you will be committed to the program and you will lose the weight. If you say 'I hope,' you won't be committed, and you will probably drop out. Today, tell yourself 'I will lose weight' and 'I will stick to the program.'"

3-Hour Timing Tip

Always carry something to read: We all have those moments of downtime—waiting for your car at the Jiffy Lube, stopping for a cup of coffee at your local coffeehouse—when it would be great to have a good book or newspaper to dive into for a few minutes.

Journal Notes

_____

_____

_____

_____

_____

_____

_____

_____

_____

_____

_____

_____

_____

_____

_____

_____

_____

_____

"Never fear the space between your dreams and reality. If you can dream it, you can make it so."

—BELVA DAVIS, JOURNALIST

DAY 14

Today's Visualization

For today's visualization, you will bump into an old boyfriend at a restaurant, someone you haven't seen in a few years. Take a few deep relaxing breathes, and then jump into the future with me—one year from today.

See yourself sitting in the restaurant with one of your girl-friends. You are both eating healthful meals. A man a few tables over keeps looking at you and then looking away. You don't recognize him at first. Eventually, he gets up and walks over to you and asks if he knows you from somewhere.

You tell him your name and he tells you his, and you make the connection. He tells you how wonderful you look. How do his comments make you feel?

Your 3-Hour Plan

1) Commit your eating times.
2) Create your custom meals from the food lists starting on page 268 or from the premade meals starting on page 283.
3) Then keep your eye on this page and check off boxes when done eating.

☐ Time: _____ **Breakfast**

Veg/Fruit
Carbs
Protein Fat

Custom Meal:
Carbs_____
Protein_____
Fat_____
Veg/Fruit_____

Premade Meal:_____

☐ Time: _____ **Snack A**

* If you weigh 200-249 lb. = double snack; 250-299 lb. = triple snack; 300+ = quadruple snack

☐ Time: _____ **Lunch**

Veg/Fruit
Carbs
Protein Fat

Custom Meal:
Carbs_____
Protein_____
Fat_____
Veg/Fruit_____

Premade Meal:_____

☐ Time: _____ **Snack B**

* If you weigh 200-249 lb. = double snack; 250-299 lb. = triple snack; 300+ = quadruple snack

☐ Time: _____ **Dinner**

Veg/Fruit
Carbs
Protein Fat

Custom Meal:
Carbs_____
Protein_____
Fat_____
Veg/Fruit_____

Premade Meal:_____

☐ Time: _____ **Treat**

_____

Water

☐ ☐ ☐ ☐ ☐ ☐ ☐ ☐

Freebie Tracker

DAY 14

"Weight loss takes a decision. When you go to work, you put on your shoes, pants, and shirt. There are no if's, and's or but's. You have to get dressed before leaving the house. You've got to approach weight loss with the same mind-set. Make a decision to eat every three hours and make it a must-do. Then, no excuse will get in your way."

3-Hour Timing Tip

Set a time limit for boring tasks: For example, when it's time to pack your snacks in the evening, limit your time spent on the chore to 20 minutes. When that time allotment is up, stop what you're doing.

Journal Notes

_____

_____

_____

_____

_____

_____

_____

_____

_____

_____

_____

_____

_____

_____

_____

_____

_____

_____

_____

_____

_____

_____

_____

_____

_____

_____

_____

_____

_____

_____

_____

_____

_____

Weigh In

My current weight is:

Height: 5'8"
Age: 36
Starting weight: 281.8 lbs.
Current weight: 261.8 lbs.
Other: Married with a teenage daughter
  from a previous marriage; works
  part-time

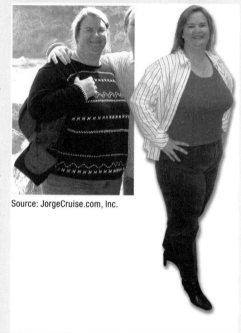

Source: JorgeCruise.com, Inc.

"Before I ran across Jorge Cruise, I was depressed and unhealthy. Our family ate whenever we could, whatever we could. Because we are busy people, we frequently ate one or two meals a day: huge, unhealthy meals, and unhealthy snacks. When I started the 3 Hour Diet™, I was surprised to realize that I had been snacking on volumes of food almost constantly in the afternoons.

"Starting this program has been one of the most healthy things I've done for myself. I've tried losing weight by exercising—even once with a great and expensive trainer. I even tried losing weight by training for and completing a marathon in 2002. I never lost much weight, and I started this program with more weight added on than ever before.

"This plan makes common sense. All of the other diets I've tried have been extreme. This program made so much sense that I worried I would feel too 'normal' on it. Today that is where I'm at, feeling normal, and losing weight gradually. Normal is a tremendously wonderful feeling for an obese person. I have not been depressed, I have not been an emotional wreck, and I haven't flung any shoes out of frustration since I started the 3-Hour Diet™. I'll hit my goal weight at some point, but in the meantime, **I have a way of life that keeps me healthy and optimistic, something I value over a size ten any and every day!**"

Victoria's Secrets to Success

> ➤ Set an alarm on your cell phone to remind yourself to eat. Set the tone to something fun like "Hallelujah" so eating can be a celebration again, not a frustration.
> ➤ Take the time to prepare in advance and make sure you have "emergency rations" in your purse or car.

"I believe that when you realize who you really are, you understand that nothing can stop you from becoming that person."

—CHRISTINE LINCOLN, AUTHOR

Today's Visualization

Today you will use the power of visualization to help fuel healthy eating choices. Today you're going to prepare a delicious salad, made with vegetables you've grown yourself in your very own garden. Close your eyes and take a few relaxing breaths, in through your nose and out through your mouth.

Imagine you've just returned home from your local garden center with your trunk full of everything you need to start your garden—fertilized soil, seedlings, transplants, shovel, hoe, watering can, and gloves. You go inside and slip on a pair of overalls, smear on some sunscreen, and place a wide-brimmed hat on your head. You look at yourself in the mirror and grin at your reflection.

You grab a water bottle from the fridge and flip on the stereo loud enough so you'll hear it outside. Feel the sun warm your cheeks as you start hoeing the soil. Your arms, strong and firm. What have you decided to plant in your garden? Tomatoes or green beans? Peppers, or perhaps a variety of herbs? Or maybe you've decided on a beautiful selection of flowers? As you dig the soil and plant each seed or transplant, concentrate on how strong your body feels. Once you've got everything planted, you sprinkle fertilizer and water over the area. You treat the garden with gentle care, giving it the nutrients it needs to grow! Picture how the garden will look in a few weeks, and then in a month. Imagine the vegetables growing ripe and delicious. What dishes will you make with the zucchini you've grown?

Your 3-Hour Plan

1) Commit your eating times.
2) Create your custom meals from the food lists starting on page 268 or from the premade meals starting on page 283.
3) Then keep your eye on this page and check off boxes when done eating.

☐ **Time:** _____ **Breakfast**

Veg/Fruit
Carbs
Protein
Fat

Custom Meal:
Carbs_____
Protein_____
Fat_____
Veg/Fruit_____

Premade Meal:_____

☐ **Time:** _____ **Snack A**

* If you weigh 200-249 lb. = double snack; 250-299 lb. = triple snack; 300+ = quadruple snack

☐ **Time:** _____ **Lunch**

Veg/Fruit
Carbs
Protein
Fat

Custom Meal:
Carbs_____
Protein_____
Fat_____
Veg/Fruit_____

Premade Meal:_____

☐ **Time:** _____ **Snack B**

* If you weigh 200-249 lb. = double snack; 250-299 lb. = triple snack; 300+ = quadruple snack

☐ **Time:** _____ **Dinner**

Veg/Fruit
Carbs
Protein
Fat

Custom Meal:
Carbs_____
Protein_____
Fat_____
Veg/Fruit_____

Premade Meal:_____

☐ **Time:** _____ **Treat**

Water

Freebie Tracker

DAY 15

3-Hour Timing Tip

*C*arry *a notebook around with you wherever you go:* Slip a small one into your purse so you can jot down thoughts that come to your mind. Or if you get the urge to eat something you shouldn't while you're on the road, you can express your feelings in your notebook instead of taking them out on a cheeseburger and fries.

Journal Notes

_____

_____

_____

_____

_____

_____

_____

_____

_____

_____

_____

_____

_____

_____

_____

_____

_____

_____

_____

_____

"We were all designed to fly!"

—DR. H. PAUL JACOBI

3

DAY 16

Today's Visualization

During today's visualization, you will imagine a whole day's worth of your favorite healthy food choices. So close your eyes and take a few deep, relaxing breaths, in through your nose and out through your mouth.

You've woken up and gotten out of bed. Now you're heading to the kitchen to prepare yourself a wholesome breakfast. What will you be eating? Will you be filling your plate with scrambled egg whites, a piece of whole-grain toast with a little butter, and an orange? Will you enjoy a cup of green tea? Decide what you will eat that will give you the energy and nutrients that your body needs to get you through the morning.

Three hours later, it's time for a snack. Will you have a cup of yogurt or some string cheese? What about for lunch? Will you join a friend for sushi and soup, or maybe head to the deli for a delicious, veggie-packed sandwich? Three hours later, you've got a dinner date. Decide which veggies will fill your plate. What else will you have? And then of course, you have a special treat, possibly a Hershey's Kiss®. Imagine yourself eating and enjoying each meal. Remember, food is fuel and your body feels so great when you give it what it needs.

Your 3-Hour Plan

1) Commit your eating times.
2) Create your custom meals from the food lists starting on page 268 or from the premade meals starting on page 283.
3) Then keep your eye on this page and check off boxes when done eating.

☐ **Time:** _____ | **Breakfast**

Veg/Fruit
Carbs
Protein
Fat

Custom Meal:
Carbs_____
Protein_____
Fat_____
Veg/Fruit_____

Premade Meal:_____

☐ **Time:** _____ | **Snack A**

---
* If you weigh 200-249 lb. = double snack; 250-299 lb. = triple snack; 300+ = quadruple snack

☐ **Time:** _____ | **Lunch**

Veg/Fruit
Carbs
Protein
Fat

Custom Meal:
Carbs_____
Protein_____
Fat_____
Veg/Fruit_____

Premade Meal:_____

☐ **Time:** _____ | **Snack B**

---
* If you weigh 200-249 lb. = double snack; 250-299 lb. = triple snack; 300+ = quadruple snack

☐ **Time:** _____ | **Dinner**

Veg/Fruit
Carbs
Protein
Fat

Custom Meal:
Carbs_____
Protein_____
Fat_____
Veg/Fruit_____

Premade Meal:_____

☐ **Time:** _____ | **Treat**

Water

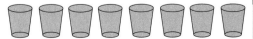

Freebie Tracker

DAY 16

JORGE-ISM

"Fat is not the problem. It's a lack of lean muscle tissue. Lean muscle tissue runs your metabolism! Overweight has everything to do with lack of muscle use!"

3-Hour Timing Tip

*P*ack all your food for the week at once: On Sunday night, or whichever night of the week precedes your work week, spend time packing all your food for the week in individual bags—one for each day. By laying everything out and packing it at once, you'll save yourself five days worth of getting the food out you need to pack and putting it away again. When it's time to leave for work in the morning, all you'll have to do is grab, a bag and head out the door!

Journal Notes

_____

_____

_____

_____

_____

_____

_____

_____

_____

_____

_____

_____

_____

_____

"If we did all the things we are capable of, we would literally astound ourselves."

—THOMAS EDISON

DAY 17

Today's Visualization

Today I want you to close your eyes. Take a few deep breaths and visualize yourself at the grocery store. You are standing in the supermarket checkout line and pick up an issue of *First for Women* magazine. You open it up and there you are, as a featured success story in a popular women's magazine. You are so excited! A huge smile appears on your face as you look at your after picture, taken only a few weeks earlier at a very special photo shoot, complete with a makeover and a stunning new hairstyle. You look truly amazing!

How eager are you to share this with everyone around you: friends, family, and coworkers, even people on the street. Do you buy more than one copy to share? How proud are you right now? How great do you feel when you realize that your story is being read by millions of people and inspiring them to take action and change their life today? Think about all the compliments and congratulations you will get and how great it will feel to know that you achieved this success.

Remember this feeling, hold onto it for a few minutes. Now jump back to the present and visualize what you must do right now to make this a reality, and before you know it you will be submitting your photos and story to us at JorgeCruise.com—you can do it!

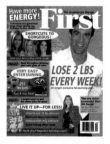

Every issue make sure to read Jorge's "Slimming Coach" column for the latest in slimming motivation.

Your 3-Hour Plan

1) Commit your eating times.
2) Create your custom meals from the food lists starting on page 268 or from the premade meals starting on page 283.
3) Then keep your eye on this page and check off boxes when done eating.

☐ **Time:** _____ | **Breakfast**

Veg/Fruit
Carbs
Protein
Fat

Custom Meal:
Carbs_____
Protein_____
Fat_____
Veg/Fruit_____

Premade Meal:_____

☐ **Time:** _____ | **Snack A**

* If you weigh 200-249 lb. = double snack; 250-299 lb. = triple snack; 300+ = quadruple snack

☐ **Time:** _____ | **Lunch**

Veg/Fruit
Carbs
Protein
Fat

Custom Meal:
Carbs_____
Protein_____
Fat_____
Veg/Fruit_____

Premade Meal:_____

☐ **Time:** _____ | **Snack B**

* If you weigh 200-249 lb. = double snack; 250-299 lb. = triple snack; 300+ = quadruple snack

☐ **Time:** _____ | **Dinner**

Veg/Fruit
Carbs
Protein
Fat

Custom Meal:
Carbs_____
Protein_____
Fat_____
Veg/Fruit_____

Premade Meal:_____

☐ **Time:** _____ | **Treat**

Water

◡ ◡ ◡ ◡ ◡ ◡ ◡ ◡

Freebie Tracker

DAY 17

3-Hour Timing Tip

*D*on't attempt to do too much at once: You may feel like Wonder Woman®, but you're not. No one is. Too many of us get caught up in the "I can do everything" trap and take on too many responsibilities, from classes to social events to taking kids to sporting events and practices. The danger of the Wonder Woman® syndrome is that you'll spread yourself too thin and not give all of your responsibilities the attention they deserve. You'll also exhaust yourself and risk becoming lazy in your healthful eating habits.

Journal Notes

_____

_____

_____

_____

_____

_____

_____

_____

_____

_____

_____

_____

_____

_____

_____

_____

"To make a great dream come true, you must first have a great dream."

—DR. HANS SELYE

Today's Visualization

L et's use visualization to help you turn a lemon into lemon-
ade, shall we? No obstacles can stand in your way. Close
your eyes and take a few deep, relaxing breaths, in through
your nose and out through your mouth. You know you can
handle any situation that comes up, you are strong and in control.

See yourself driving home from the grocery store with a
backseat full of healthy, nutritious food. Hear yourself happily
singing along to your favorite song on the radio. Suddenly, you
hear a "clunk, clunk, clunk" sound as your car begins to
bounce around. It's a flat tire! Instead of panicking, you calmly
steer your car to the side of the road and turn on your hazard
lights. Carefully you open your door and get out.

See the look on your face as you assess the situation and
then go to your trunk and retrieve the spare tire, car jack, and
lug wrench. See yourself removing the hubcap, loosening the
lug nuts, and positioning the jack. You use strong, solid, even
strokes on the jack and up your car goes! You remove the flat
tire and hoist it back in your trunk, install the spare, replace
the lug nuts, lower your car, replace the hubcap, and then
you're on your way. No problem! How do you feel knowing
that you can overcome any obstacle that comes your way?

Your 3-Hour Plan

1) Commit your eating times.
2) Create your custom meals from the food lists starting on page 268 or from the premade meals starting on page 283.
3) Then keep your eye on this page and check off boxes when done eating.

☐ **Time:** _____ **Breakfast**

Veg/Fruit
Carbs
Protein   Fat

Custom Meal:
Carbs_____
Protein_____
Fat_____
Veg/Fruit_____

Premade Meal:_____

☐ **Time:** _____ **Snack A**

* If you weigh 200-249 lb. = double snack; 250-299 lb. = triple snack; 300+ = quadruple snack

☐ **Time:** _____ **Lunch**

Veg/Fruit
Carbs
Protein   Fat

Custom Meal:
Carbs_____
Protein_____
Fat_____
Veg/Fruit_____

Premade Meal:_____

☐ **Time:** _____ **Snack B**

* If you weigh 200-249 lb. = double snack; 250-299 lb. = triple snack; 300+ = quadruple snack

☐ **Time:** _____ **Dinner**

Veg/Fruit
Carbs
Protein   Fat

Custom Meal:
Carbs_____
Protein_____
Fat_____
Veg/Fruit_____

Premade Meal:_____

☐ **Time:** _____ **Treat**

Water

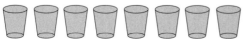

Freebie Tracker

DAY 18

JORGE-ISM

"Learn the difference between nutritional hunger and emotional hunger. Emotional hunger leads to emotional eating. Emotional eating is the #1 obstacle that stops people from getting the results from weight loss."

3-Hour Timing Tip

Stop procrastinating: When you put something off until to-morrow, you lose today forever. Procrastination is the easy way out; it has no benefits. You will not do something better if you put it off until the last minute.

Journal Notes

_____

_____

_____

_____

_____

_____

_____

_____

_____

_____

_____

_____

_____

_____

_____

_____

_____

_____

"You have to have faith and believe in yourself."

—GAIL DEVERES, ATHLETE

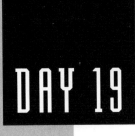

DAY 19

Today's Visualization

For today's visualization, you will use the power of your mind to help you solve problems that might have led to emotional eating in the past. Close your eyes and take a few relaxing breaths, in through your nose and out through your mouth. Today you will use visualization to help you overcome the urge to eat when you encounter difficult people. Take a few moments to relax by taking a few deep breaths. Feel each exhalation relax you more and more deeply. Once you are fully relaxed, you are ready to begin.

Imagine someone with whom you may be having some personal conflict. It might be your spouse or your child or someone at work. Bring the image of that person into your mind. Then I want you to imagine having a positive interaction with that person. Start with some small talk. See yourself confronting this person about what is bothering you. See yourself calmly, nicely, and succinctly voicing your concerns, keeping the focus on how this person makes you feel. See this person respond positively, perhaps by saying, "I didn't know you felt this way." And then imagine a positive end to the encounter. You will soon find that if you mentally see yourself confronting your problems, you won't feel so much stress or anxiety when you try to solve them in real life!

Your 3-Hour Plan

1) Commit your eating times.
2) Create your custom meals from the food lists starting on page 268 or from the premade meals starting on page 283.
3) Then keep your eye on this page and check off boxes when done eating.

☐ **Time:** _____ **Breakfast**

Veg/Fruit
Carbs
Protein   Fat

Custom Meal:
Carbs_____
Protein_____
Fat_____
Veg/Fruit_____
Premade Meal:_____

☐ **Time:** _____ **Snack A**

* If you weigh 200-249 lb. = double snack; 250-299 lb. = triple snack; 300+ = quadruple snack

☐ **Time:** _____ **Lunch**

Veg/Fruit
Carbs
Protein   Fat

Custom Meal:
Carbs_____
Protein_____
Fat_____
Veg/Fruit_____
Premade Meal:_____

☐ **Time:** _____ **Snack B**

* If you weigh 200-249 lb. = double snack; 250-299 lb. = triple snack; 300+ = quadruple snack

☐ **Time:** _____ **Dinner**

Veg/Fruit
Carbs
Protein   Fat

Custom Meal:
Carbs_____
Protein_____
Fat_____
Veg/Fruit_____
Premade Meal:_____

☐ **Time:** _____ **Treat**

Water

☐ ☐ ☐ ☐ ☐ ☐ ☐ ☐

Freebie Tracker

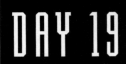

DAY 19

3-Hour Timing Tip

Break out of the perfectionism trap: Don't get me wrong—doing things to the best of your ability is a good rule of thumb. But some people take this motto to an unhealthy extreme and get bogged down in unnecessary details. Or they become control freaks and have to do everything themselves instead of accepting help when it's available. Learn to step away from a task when it's done well enough.

Journal Notes

_____

_____

_____

_____

_____

_____

_____

_____

_____

_____

_____

_____

_____

_____

_____

_____

_____

"Set your goals high, and
don't stop till you get there."

—BO JACKSON, ATHLETE

DAY 20

Today's Visualization

Many of my clients tell me that they are most likely to overeat when they feel worthless or "not good enough." Today's visualization will help you to overcome such feelings. Today you will cultivate your inner self-love. Close your eyes and take a few deep, relaxing breaths, in through your nose and out through your mouth. Once you feel completely relaxed, you are ready to begin.

See yourself doing something that you do everyday. Perhaps you are at work. Perhaps you are at the grocery store. Perhaps you are out with friends or with your children. Try to see yourself through the eyes of someone else, someone who really cares about you such as a close friend, spouse, or one of your children. This person really cares about you and admires you. Feel the same admiration that this person feels as you watch yourself through your friend's, spouse's, or child's eyes. Try to see all of the good qualities about yourself that they see every day.

Watch yourself from afar as your loved ones walk up to you and tell you how much they love and admire you. Watch your expression as they tell you about your good qualities. What do they say? Now imagine more and more people coming into the room and staring at you with the same love and admiration of your loved one. As the room fills with people, they begin to applaud, clapping for you!

Your 3-Hour Plan

1) Commit your eating times.
2) Create your custom meals from the food lists starting on page 268 or from the premade meals starting on page 283.
3) Then keep your eye on this page and check off boxes when done eating.

☐ **Time:** _____ **Breakfast**

Veg/Fruit
Carbs
Protein   Fat

Custom Meal:
Carbs_____
Protein_____
Fat_____
Veg/Fruit_____

Premade Meal:_____

☐ **Time:** _____ **Snack A**

_____
* If you weigh 200-249 lb. = double snack; 250-299 lb. = triple snack; 300+ = quadruple snack

☐ **Time:** _____ **Lunch**

Veg/Fruit
Carbs
Protein   Fat

Custom Meal:
Carbs_____
Protein_____
Fat_____
Veg/Fruit_____

Premade Meal:_____

☐ **Time:** _____ **Snack B**

_____
* If you weigh 200-249 lb. = double snack; 250-299 lb. = triple snack; 300+ = quadruple snack

☐ **Time:** _____ **Dinner**

Veg/Fruit
Carbs
Protein   Fat

Custom Meal:
Carbs_____
Protein_____
Fat_____
Veg/Fruit_____

Premade Meal:_____

☐ **Time:** _____ **Treat**

_____

Water

Freebie Tracker

DAY 20

"You must deal with emotional eating. If you don't, food will always be a comforter for you. Eating when you're not hungry is emotional eating. You don't want to do that. This self-sabotage will get you every single time. Use the power of people and connections to replace emotional eating."

3-Hour Timing Tip

Solve problems before they start: If you address upfront small issues that you foresee growing into larger problems later on, you'll stop a big problem before it starts. For example, if you know you have a big presentation to do at work that may involve some controversial topics, run those topics by your supervisor as you include them, so you don't have to do the whole thing over at the end. Same goes for similar situations in your personal life.

Journal Notes

_____

_____

_____

_____

_____

_____

_____

_____

_____

_____

_____

_____

_____

_____

"If you can believe it,
the mind can achieve it."

—RONNIE LOTT, ATHLETE

3

DAY 21

Today's Visualization

Today you will use the power of visualization to help overcome negative feelings that can lead to overeating. You can use this visualization any time you feel a negative mood coming on. Use it whenever you find a negative emotion causing you to think of food.

Start by relaxing with a few deep breaths. Allow each exhalation to bring you to a deeper and deeper state of relaxation. Once you feel deeply relaxed, you are ready to begin.

Notice the state of your mind. Are you feeling any negative emotions? Do you feel angry, sad, depressed, anxious, or fearful? Each time you exhale, see yourself releasing these negative feelings out of your body. See your breath literally blow them away! Then, each time you inhale, visualize yourself breathing in positive emotions such as love, compassion, joy, and peace. With each breath, exchange a negative emotion for a positive one, and feel your body begin to vibrate with positive emotions!

Your 3-Hour Plan

1) Commit your eating times.
2) Create your custom meals from the food lists starting on page 268 or from the premade meals starting on page 283.
3) Then keep your eye on this page and check off boxes when done eating.

☐ **Time:** _____ **Breakfast**

Veg/Fruit
Carbs
Protein   Fat

Custom Meal:
Carbs_____
Protein_____
Fat_____
Veg/Fruit_____

Premade Meal:_____

☐ **Time:** _____ **Snack A**

---

* If you weigh 200-249 lb. = double snack; 250-299 lb. = triple snack; 300+ = quadruple snack

☐ **Time:** _____ **Lunch**

Veg/Fruit
Carbs
Protein   Fat

Custom Meal:
Carbs_____
Protein_____
Fat_____
Veg/Fruit_____

Premade Meal:_____

☐ **Time:** _____ **Snack B**

---

* If you weigh 200-249 lb. = double snack; 250-299 lb. = triple snack; 300+ = quadruple snack

☐ **Time:** _____ **Dinner**

Veg/Fruit
Carbs
Protein   Fat

Custom Meal:
Carbs_____
Protein_____
Fat_____
Veg/Fruit_____

Premade Meal:_____

☐ **Time:** _____ **Treat**

Water

🥛 🥛 🥛 🥛 🥛 🥛 🥛 🥛

Freebie Tracker

DAY 21

JORGE-ISM

"Don't be disrespectful to your body. Your body won't be happy and you won't be happy. You need to be a friend to yourself, be nurturing to yourself, and be loving to yourself."

3-Hour Timing Tip

arry emergency rations with you: You never know when you'll find yourself stuck in a situation—such as a business meeting—when it's not appropriate to eat. Encountering such a situation when it's the time of day for a meal or snack doesn't have to derail your success on the 3-Hour Diet™. Keep a supply of drinkable yogurts and meal replacement shakes or bars in your purse, desk, or office fridge. Then, when you know a meeting will run over your snack or meal time, you'll be prepared to eat on the go.

Journal Notes

_____

_____

_____

_____

_____

_____

_____

_____

_____

_____

_____

_____

_____

_____

_____

_____

_____

_____

_____

Weigh In

My current weight is:

Heigh 5'3"
Age: 62
Starting Weight: 203 lbs.
Current weight: 163 lbs
Other: Married mother of 3, grandmother
of 8; works as a pastor and part-time
writer

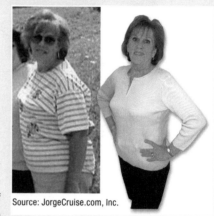

Source: JorgeCruise.com, Inc.

"Before the 3-Hour Diet™, I had lost control over my eating (never mind exercising). As a pastor, I was always in front of people; this made it even harder because I thought they would be judging me (they weren't). I was not only dealing with not being in control of my weight, but I was dealing with the guilt of being a bad example to others.

"After the birth of my second child, I gained weight and began a 40-year battle of the bulge. I became consumed with it. I tried every diet gimmick known to man, and then some. They all worked for while. But nothing changed my thinking, or my weight, until God answered my prayer of desperation and I discovered the 3-Hour Diet™.

"**A year later and 40 pounds lighter, I still can't believe what I see in the mirror. All I ever wanted to be was a normal size, and now I do not have to go in the plus-size stores for clothes (which I hated with a passion). I eat better and feel better than I did twenty years ago.** My back doesn't hurt. I am not always taking painkillers for headaches. An added blessing was when I got a report from my doctor that my osteoporosis test was normal after being on medication for years. This 'old' lady in the mirror can now lift 12-pound weights, and can do things she never did before!

"When people ask what happened (which they always do) I love to tell them that what God did for me through the Jorge Cruise's method, He can do for them. In my case, God did save the best for last. Thank you, Jorge!"

Fran's Secrets to Success

- ➤ Shop with a list for the right foods to avoid buying too many "goodies."
- ➤ Always keep a good selection of healthy and fun foods in the house.
- ➤ Plan what to eat when out.
- ➤ Drink lots of flavored seltzer with meals to prevent overeating.

"I don't ever look back.
I look forward."

—STEFFI GRAF, ATHLETE

Today's Visualization

Today is your good friend's birthday and you've invited her over for a healthy and delicious gourmet dinner. Are you ready to get cooking? Close your eyes and take a few relaxing breaths, in through your nose and out through your mouth.

You carefully planned the menu earlier in the week and purchased everything you need. What will you be serving as an appetizer? Perhaps a yummy hummus dip with crisp, fresh veggies? What will be your main dish? You might choose a savory roast chicken, steamy veggie fajitas, or a delicate, poached salmon. Will you serve a beautiful green salad, tossed with a variety of fresh, colorful veggies and dressed with your own homemade vinaigrette? Will you serve steamed asparagus or broccoli on the side? And don't forget the birthday cake!

You hear the doorbell ring just as you finish chopping the last few veggies for the salad. See yourself opening the door and greeting your friend with a big birthday hug. As she follows you into the kitchen she comments on how delicious everything smells. You lead her to the dining table, which you've set with your best dishes and decorated with a vase full of her favorite flowers. You pour two glasses of wine and say a toast to her birthday. See yourself serving each dish as the birthday girl oohs and ahhs. Enjoy each bite and stop eating when you're satisfied, not overly full.

When the dinner is cleared, you dim the lights and bring out the cake. She blows out the candles and you each savor a delectable slice. As she prepares to leave, you box up the leftovers for her to enjoy the next day. She gives you a big hug and says, "Thank you so much! This really made me feel special. You are a great friend."

Your 3-Hour Plan

1) Commit your eating times.
2) Create your custom meals from the food lists starting on page 268 or from the premade meals starting on page 283.
3) Then keep your eye on this page and check off boxes when done eating.

☐ **Time:** _____ | **Breakfast**

Veg/Fruit
Carbs
Protein   Fat

Custom Meal:
Carbs_____
Protein_____
Fat_____
Veg/Fruit_____

Premade Meal:_____

☐ **Time:** _____ | **Snack A**

* If you weigh 200-249 lb. = double snack; 250-299 lb. = triple snack; 300+ = quadruple snack

☐ **Time:** _____ | **Lunch**

Veg/Fruit
Carbs
Protein   Fat

Custom Meal:
Carbs_____
Protein_____
Fat_____
Veg/Fruit_____

Premade Meal:_____

☐ **Time:** _____ | **Snack B**

* If you weigh 200-249 lb. = double snack; 250-299 lb. = triple snack; 300+ = quadruple snack

☐ **Time:** _____ | **Dinner**

Veg/Fruit
Carbs
Protein   Fat

Custom Meal:
Carbs_____
Protein_____
Fat_____
Veg/Fruit_____

Premade Meal:_____

☐ **Time:** _____ | **Treat**

Water

Freebie Tracker

DAY 22

3-Hour Timing Tip

Schedule appointments with yourself: Whether it's to actually finish something you've been meaning to get done, like cleaning out the basement, or to fit in some much-needed relaxation time, set appointments with yourself as you would with friends or colleagues. "Tuesday night, 7 p.m.—time to give myself a manicure." Or "Thursday morning, pack all my meals for the next week." And *keep* them.

Journal Notes

"When you feel good about yourself, others will feel good about you, too."

—JAKE (BODY BY JAKE) STEINFELD

DAY 23

Today's Visualization

Today we will again jump into the future, to Thanksgiving Day after you have reached your goal weight. Close your eyes and take a few relaxing breaths, in through your nose and out through your mouth. See all of the wonderful, delicious foods on the table. Notice how you feel. Did you eat 3 hours ago, according to plan? Yes, you did.

You don't feel famished, as you have in the past. You don't notice any cravings. You feel completely in control. Take your plate and fill it up with healthful options, dishing up reasonable portions. What did you put on your plate and how does it look?

As you begin to eat, notice that you still feel in control. Chew your food and taste every bite. Notice how much more slowly you eat when you are not famished. Notice how much more you enjoy your meal. Once you finish, place your napkin over your plate. Notice how you feel satisfied, but not stuffed. Others around the table are unbuttoning their pants and loosening their belts, but you feel completely comfortable. Congratulations!

Your 3-Hour Plan

1) Commit your eating times.
2) Create your custom meals from the food lists starting on page 268 or from the premade meals starting on page 283.
3) Then keep your eye on this page and check off boxes when done eating.

☐ Time: _____ **Breakfast**

Veg/Fruit
Carbs
Protein
Fat

Custom Meal:
Carbs_____
Protein_____
Fat_____
Veg/Fruit_____

Premade Meal:_____

☐ Time: _____ **Snack A**

---

* If you weigh 200-249 lb. = double snack; 250-299 lb. = triple snack; 300+ = quadruple snack

☐ Time: _____ **Lunch**

Veg/Fruit
Carbs
Protein
Fat

Custom Meal:
Carbs_____
Protein_____
Fat_____
Veg/Fruit_____

Premade Meal:_____

☐ Time: _____ **Snack B**

---

* If you weigh 200-249 lb. = double snack; 250-299 lb. = triple snack; 300+ = quadruple snack

☐ Time: _____ **Dinner**

Veg/Fruit
Carbs
Protein
Fat

Custom Meal:
Carbs_____
Protein_____
Fat_____
Veg/Fruit_____

Premade Meal:_____

☐ Time: _____ **Treat**

Water

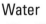

Freebie Tracker

DAY 23

"Some of my clients forget to eat every three hours. My suggestion to them and you is to set an alarm to beep every three hours, or if at work set their computer calendar to beep at them. Make sure you find a way to remind yourself to eat every three hours."

3-Hour Timing Tip

Watch your socializing time: We all love to spend time chatting at the office or on the phone when we get home, but five minutes here and there can add up to an hour once the day is through. Make sure your socializing time is spent wisely and frugally, and you'll be surprised at how much time you save.

Journal Notes

"If you don't ask,
you don't get."

—MOHANDAS GANDHI

DAY 24

Today's Visualization

Today you have been invited to speak at your son or daughter's school. Close your eyes and take a few relaxing breaths, in through your nose and out through your mouth. In the past, you might have been embarrassed to speak in front of your child's class, explaining what you do for a living. You might have felt that the other children would tease your child.

Today, however, is long after you've reached your goal weight. You look and feel fantastic. See yourself walking into the classroom and sitting down in front. Hear yourself telling the children about what you do for a living. See the smiles on their faces as they listen with rapt attention. As you talk, take a glimpse at your child. See how proud he is of you.

As you get up to leave, your son or daughter runs up to hug you. How great does that feel?

Your 3-Hour Plan

1) Commit your eating times.
2) Create your custom meals from the food lists starting on page 268 or from the premade meals starting on page 283.
3) Then keep your eye on this page and check off boxes when done eating.

☐ **Time:** _____ **Breakfast**

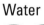

Veg/Fruit
Carbs
Protein   Fat

Custom Meal:
Carbs_____
Protein_____
Fat_____
Veg/Fruit_____

Premade Meal:_____

☐ **Time:** _____ **Snack A**

---

* If you weigh 200-249 lb. = double snack; 250-299 lb. = triple snack; 300+ = quadruple snack

☐ **Time:** _____ **Lunch**

Veg/Fruit
Carbs
Protein   Fat

Custom Meal:
Carbs_____
Protein_____
Fat_____
Veg/Fruit_____

Premade Meal:_____

☐ **Time:** _____ **Snack B**

---

* If you weigh 200-249 lb. = double snack; 250-299 lb. = triple snack; 300+ = quadruple snack

☐ **Time:** _____ **Dinner**

Veg/Fruit
Carbs
Protein   Fat

Custom Meal:
Carbs_____
Protein_____
Fat_____
Veg/Fruit_____

Premade Meal:_____

☐ **Time:** _____ **Treat**

Water

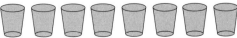

Freebie Tracker

DAY 24

"You are going to be eating with the goal of keeping your body firm, strong, and sexy. To do that, you must preserve lean muscle tissue, which requires you eat every three hours."

3-Hour Timing Tip

*L*ive in the here and now: Future goals are very important. After all, they help drive us. But in order to get to those goals, you must concentrate on what you're doing right now. And living in the now helps you stop and smell the roses and say, "This moment is wonderful. I'm really enjoying myself right now"—which is important for maintaining a positive attitude.

Journal Notes

_____

_____

_____

_____

_____

_____

_____

_____

_____

_____

_____

_____

_____

_____

_____

_____

_____

*"Per ardua ad astra.
[By striving we reach
the stars.]"*

—ROYAL AIR FORCE MOTTO

DAY 25

Today's Visualization

Today you are going to use visualization to help build your inner gratitude. Once you build gratitude, you'll more easily be able to handle any negative emotions that may have led to overeating in the past. Close your eyes and take a few deep, relaxing breaths. Every time you exhale, allow your body to grow more and more relaxed. Once you feel completely relaxed, you are ready to start.

Reflect on your good qualities and on how you affect others in your life. Are you a good friend or mother? What good things have you done in your life? You might remember the birth of your child or a good deed you did for someone in need. Recall a time when you were instrumental in making someone else happy. Try to recall every detail. For the next few moments, continue to dwell on those details when you lived up to your expectations for yourself. Realize that you have done more good than bad in this world. Allow yourself to feel grateful for yourself. Allow this gratitude to grow in your heart.

Your 3-Hour Plan

1) Commit your eating times.
2) Create your custom meals from the food lists starting on page 268 or from the premade meals starting on page 283.
3) Then keep your eye on this page and check off boxes when done eating.

☐ **Time:** _____ | **Breakfast**

Veg/Fruit
Carbs
Protein Fat

Custom Meal:
Carbs_____
Protein_____
Fat_____
Veg/Fruit_____

Premade Meal:_____

☐ **Time:** _____ | **Snack A**

* If you weigh 200-249 lb. = double snack; 250-299 lb. = triple snack; 300+ = quadruple snack

☐ **Time:** _____ | **Lunch**

Veg/Fruit
Carbs
Protein Fat

Custom Meal:
Carbs_____
Protein_____
Fat_____
Veg/Fruit_____

Premade Meal:_____

☐ **Time:** _____ | **Snack B**

* If you weigh 200-249 lb. = double snack; 250-299 lb. = triple snack; 300+ = quadruple snack

☐ **Time:** _____ | **Dinner**

Veg/Fruit
Carbs
Protein Fat

Custom Meal:
Carbs_____
Protein_____
Fat_____
Veg/Fruit_____

Premade Meal:_____

☐ **Time:** _____ | **Treat**

Water

Freebie Tracker

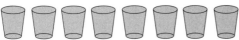

DAY 25

"Make this plan enjoyable. You're going to do this long-term and be healthy for a lifetime!"

3-Hour Timing Tip

Get organized: You can't think clearly if your surroundings are cluttered. A messy desk or kitchen will hinder your ability to complete tasks like bill paying or meal preparation.

Journal Notes

_____

_____

_____

_____

_____

_____

_____

_____

_____

_____

_____

_____

_____

_____

_____

_____

_____

_____

_____

_____

"Wheresoever you go,
go with all your heart."

—CONFUCIUS

DAY 26

Today's Visualization

Imagine yourself one evening in the future. Close your eyes and take a few relaxing breaths, in through your nose and out through your mouth. Your neighbors have invited you over for a "dessert party." You know the party will be full of cheesecake, cookies, brownies, and other treats. Notice how in control you feel. In the past you might have declined to attend such a party, feeling you would overindulge. Today, however, you feel completely in control.

See yourself walk into the party. Various people from the neighborhood are there. Many walk up to you and tell you how great you look. They ask how you lost the weight, and you tell them.

Walk over to the dessert table. Scan the table, still feeling in control. Pick out a small treat. Slowly eat it, savoring every bite. Then see yourself walk away from the table with control. Congratulations!

Your 3-Hour Plan

1) Commit your eating times.
2) Create your custom meals from the food lists starting on page 268 or from the premade meals starting on page 283.
3) Then keep your eye on this page and check off boxes when done eating.

☐ Time: _____ **Breakfast**

Veg/Fruit
Carbs
Protein   Fat

Custom Meal:
Carbs_____
Protein_____
Fat_____
Veg/Fruit_____

Premade Meal:_____

☐ Time: _____ **Snack A**

* If you weigh 200-249 lb. = double snack; 250-299 lb. = triple snack; 300+ = quadruple snack

☐ Time: _____ **Lunch**

Veg/Fruit
Carbs
Protein   Fat

Custom Meal:
Carbs_____
Protein_____
Fat_____
Veg/Fruit_____

Premade Meal:_____

☐ Time: _____ **Snack B**

* If you weigh 200-249 lb. = double snack; 250-299 lb. = triple snack; 300+ = quadruple snack

☐ Time: _____ **Dinner**

Veg/Fruit
Carbs
Protein   Fat

Custom Meal:
Carbs_____
Protein_____
Fat_____
Veg/Fruit_____

Premade Meal:_____

☐ Time: _____ **Treat**

Water

Freebie Tracker

DAY 26

3-Hour Timing Tip

Don't exhaust yourself: Whether you're paying bills or planning your meals for the week, recognize when you need to take a break from something. If you're gazing out the window or balancing your ruler on your desk, or worst of all—thinking about the leftover pizza you have in the fridge—take a five-minute break. But don't go to the fridge!

Journal Notes

_____

_____

_____

_____

_____

_____

_____

_____

_____

_____

_____

_____

_____

_____

_____

_____

_____

_____

"Yesterday is but a dream,
and tomorrow is only a vision,
but today well lived makes
every yesterday a dream of
happiness and every
tomorrow a vision of hope."

—UNKNOWN

DAY 27

Today's Visualization

Today, let's again take a trip well into the future, long after you've reached your goal weight. Close your eyes and take a few relaxing breaths, in through your nose and out through your mouth. Today you are going to see yourself at the pinnacle of life, living life to your potential.

Imagine yourself at home five years from now. You've reached your goal weight and have maintained it for more than four years. Your career and family life are perfect and you live in the home of your dreams. Look around you. What are you surrounded by? Who is in the room with you? What do you look like? How do you feel?

Take in all of the sights, sounds, smells, and sensations of your perfect life. You got to this place because you set goals and then achieved them. You now have everything you will ever need and you are completely content. Treasure this sensation before releasing the visualization of the future. You've earned it!

Your 3-Hour Plan

1) Commit your eating times.
2) Create your custom meals from the food lists starting on page 268 or from the premade meals starting on page 283.
3) Then keep your eye on this page and check off boxes when done eating.

☐ Time:	Breakfast

Custom Meal:
Carbs_____
Protein_____
Fat_____
Veg/Fruit_____

Premade Meal:_____

Veg/Fruit — Carbs — Protein — Fat

☐ Time:	Snack A

* If you weigh 200-249 lb. = double snack; 250-299 lb. = triple snack; 300+ = quadruple snack

☐ Time:	Lunch

Custom Meal:
Carbs_____
Protein_____
Fat_____
Veg/Fruit_____

Premade Meal:_____

Veg/Fruit — Carbs — Protein — Fat

☐ Time:	Snack B

* If you weigh 200-249 lb. = double snack; 250-299 lb. = triple snack; 300+ = quadruple snack

☐ Time:	Dinner

Custom Meal:
Carbs_____
Protein_____
Fat_____
Veg/Fruit_____

Premade Meal:_____

Veg/Fruit — Carbs — Protein — Fat

☐ Time:	Treat

Water

☐ ☐ ☐ ☐ ☐ ☐ ☐ ☐

Freebie Tracker

DAY 27

3-Hour Timing Tip

Get the timing right: Get to know your natural rhythms. If you're most energetic in the morning, try to get as much done as you can then. Make sure you do the things that require the most concentration when you're most alert.

Journal Notes

_____

_____

_____

_____

_____

_____

_____

_____

_____

_____

_____

_____

_____

_____

_____

_____

_____

"Life is a pure flame, and
we live by an invisible
sun within us."

—SIR THOMAS BROWNE

DAY 28

Today's Visualization

Today I want you to imagine yourself doing something you never before dreamed possible. Perhaps it's something you've put off or decided not to do because of your weight. Perhaps you've always wanted to wear a bikini to the beach or go to a water park with your family, but have resisted because you thought people would stare. Whatever it is for you—and it will be slightly different for each of you—I want you to call to mind an activity that you've always wanted to do—but haven't. Close your eyes and take a few relaxing breaths, in through your nose and out through your mouth.

Then, I want you to see yourself doing it. See every detail. Take in every sight, sound, smell, and sensation. Relish the knowledge that you can do anything you set your mind to. You've reached your goal!

Your 3-Hour Plan

1) Commit your eating times.
2) Create your custom meals from the food lists starting on page 268 or from the premade meals starting on page 283.
3) Then keep your eye on this page and check off boxes when done eating.

☐ Time: _____ **Breakfast**

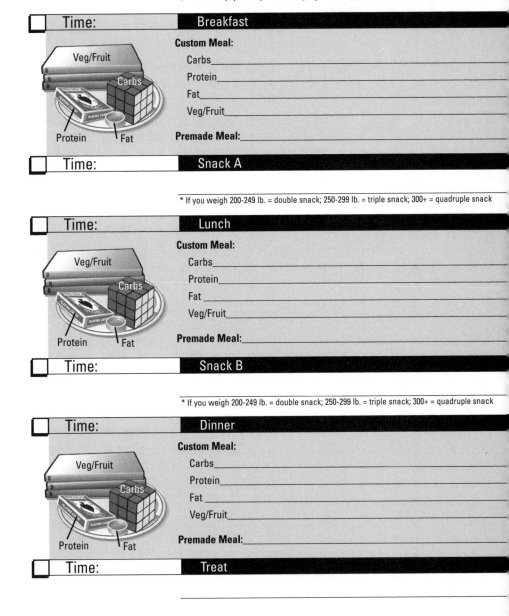

Veg/Fruit
Carbs
Protein Fat

Custom Meal:
Carbs_____
Protein_____
Fat_____
Veg/Fruit_____

Premade Meal:_____

☐ Time: _____ **Snack A**

* If you weigh 200-249 lb. = double snack; 250-299 lb. = triple snack; 300+ = quadruple snack

☐ Time: _____ **Lunch**

Veg/Fruit
Carbs
Protein Fat

Custom Meal:
Carbs_____
Protein_____
Fat_____
Veg/Fruit_____

Premade Meal:_____

☐ Time: _____ **Snack B**

* If you weigh 200-249 lb. = double snack; 250-299 lb. = triple snack; 300+ = quadruple snack

☐ Time: _____ **Dinner**

Veg/Fruit
Carbs
Protein Fat

Custom Meal:
Carbs_____
Protein_____
Fat_____
Veg/Fruit_____

Premade Meal:_____

☐ Time: _____ **Treat**

Water

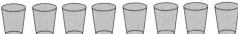

Freebie Tracker

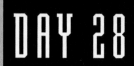

DAY 28

JORGE-ISM

"The power of support can help you overcome emotional eating. If you have a network of friends, you can turn to them instead of the fridge or cupboard."

3-Hour Timing Tip

*C*onstantly ask yourself what you can be doing to move toward your goals: Become aware of how you waste time. Ask yourself, "Would I pay myself for what I'm doing right now?" You'd be surprised at how much time you spend doing things you *wouldn't* pay yourself for.

Journal Notes

_____

_____

_____

_____

_____

_____

_____

_____

_____

_____

_____

_____

_____

_____

_____

_____

_____

_____

_____

_____

_____

_____

_____

_____

_____

_____

_____

_____

_____

_____

_____

_____

_____

Weigh In

My current weight is:

Congratulations! Now that you have finished the first 28 days, stop and celebrate your success and all that you have achieved. In the next chapter I will explain how to continue the plan, along with tips on maintenance, once you reach your goal.

Height: 5' 10"
Age: 53
Starting weight: 228 lbs.
Current weight: 188 lbs.
Other: A retired Naval Officer working
a second career in Information
Technology; married with three
grandchildren.

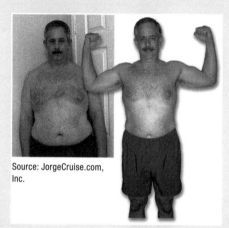

Source: JorgeCruise.com, Inc.

"Before the 3-Hour Diet™ I was ashamed that I had let myself get so out of shape! I was embarrassed at how I looked and was not comfortable in my clothes. Now, after being on Jorge's program, I am comfortable with myself, I fit into my clothes, my wife loves how I look, and I can look in the mirror at my slimmer body and feel good about how I look. I am more confident at work because I feel better about myself.

"I've succeeded on the program by following a set routine. Each day I eat breakfast at around 7:00 a.m., a snack at 10:00 a.m., lunch at 1:00 p.m., a snack at 4:00 p.m. and dinner at around 7:00 p.m. My favorite snacks are my trail mix and yogurt cups. This works for me. I never feel deprived.

"I was raised thinking that I had to finish everything on my plate. We had meat, potatoes, salad, and bread with every evening meal. Finally, with Jorge's plan, I was able to break that emotional bond I had with food and not worry about finishing all that was on my plate. Now, once I feel full, I stop eating even if there is still food on my plate. What a relief. **It did not take me long to realize that I could eat my fill, feel full, and still stay on Jorge's plan. I lost weight doing it this way and I love the results!"**

Paul's Secrets to Success

➤ Prioritize! Prioritize! Prioritize! Look at what you have to do for the day, week, month, and prioritize those tasks.
➤ Feel good about yourself.
➤ When you get the urge to eat, ask yourself whether that urge is based on true hunger or an emotional need.

3-HOUR DIET™ MAINTENANCE PLAN: HOW TO LOSE MORE OR KEEP IT OFF

efore I started the 3-Hour Diet™ I was experiencing more and more pain with my knees, extreme heartburn, and poor sleep. I would frequently feel famished when I came home from work, and couldn't function until I had eaten something. I was also constantly fatigued and had to take naps in between my tasks at home. Now, I no longer need or require daily naps. I am able to hike seven to ten miles and can carry around 35 pounds on my back. And, yes, now I love seeing myself in the mirror every morning."

—SANDY COLÓN—LOST 37 POUNDS

Congratulations for successfully completing the 28-day program! By now you should have lost about 8 pounds, enough to firmly plant you on the road to success. You've worked hard over these past 28 days, establishing healthful habits that will carry you for the rest of your life time, but you are not done yet.

The 3-Hour Solution

Your maintenance plan will help you to

- Continue to lose two pounds a week until you reach your weight loss goal
- Keep the weight off long-term
- Maintain your new eating habits for a lifetime

Perhaps you've met your goal weight, or perhaps you'd like to lose even more. Either way, in this chapter, you will find the information you need to stick with the 3-Hour Diet™ for life. Even if you have reached your goal weight, you must continue with the 3-Hour Diet™. This is critical to your long-term success. In order to keep the weight off, you must continue with the healthy habits that caused you to lose weight in the first place. Resort to your old ways of eating and the weight will steadily creep back on.

So promise yourself that you will continue your healthy habits. Think of the initial 28-day plan as a kick-start program to a new you. Think of this maintenance plan as the map you will use to take that new you on a journey that will last a lifetime!

Want to Lose More?

If you want to lose more weight, the plan is simple. Just continue what you've been doing for the past 28 days. Follow the same meal plan you've been following, either choosing sample meals from chapter 13 or creating your own custom meals by using the 3-Hour Plate™.

Each of your meals will consist of the same number of calories as before. You'll consume 400 calories at each of your three daily meals, 100 calories at each of your two snacks, and 50 calories for your after-dinner treat. I encourage you to keep track of your meals and plan for them using some type of log, just like the planner you used for the first 28 days of the program. Writing down what you will eat ahead of time will help you plan for each meal, ensuring your success.

To log your meals, you have a number of options. You can continue to cycle through the pages you've already written in for your 28-day planner, following the meal plans you've already designed. If you'd like more variety, however, you can also use our online planners from www.JorgeCruise .com.

It's that simple. Just continue doing what you've been doing and the weight will come off. Remember:

- Weigh in every Sunday. This will help keep you motivated and allow you to track your success.
- Write your meals in your logbook or planner.
- Stay in touch with your support network. They'll help you stay motivated.

A word about plateaus

I encourage you to weigh in every Sunday. However, know that from time to time, you may experience a week or two when you fail to lose weight. Don't panic. A short-term plateau can happen for a variety of reasons, including the following:

You're menstruating. Most women retain water and, therefore, gain a pound or two during that time of the month. Don't sweat this. Once your period ends, you'll step back on the scale to find that you really did continue to lose fat. Occasionally, I hear from women who struggle to stick with their eating plan during that time of the month. If you backslide and eat a little bit more—say, having a larger snack than usual—just get back on the program as soon as you can. Don't beat yourself up over it. Guilt will only lead to emotional eating.

You're taking a new medication. Certain medications, such as steroids, some heart meds, and birth control pills, can cause water retention, which will boost your weight on the scale. Others, such as certain antidepressants, can boost appetite and slow your metabolism, triggering weight gain. In many cases, simply switching to a different brand or type will solve the problem, so talk to your doctor.

You're consuming too much salt. Sodium can cause water retention. Although this isn't fat gain, it is demotivating to step on the scale

Height: 5'7½"
Age: 40
Starting Weight: 207 lbs.
Current Weight: 130 lbs.
Other: Married 17 years with twins (a boy and a girl); works part-time at an elementary school.

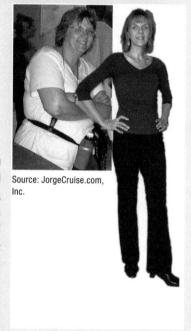

"Last August 2003 after a long vacation in Florida with my husband and 13-year-old twins, I could no longer look at myself in a photo let alone a mirror. One morning I woke up to my favorite show *Good Morning America* and there Jorge was talking with Diane Sawyer alongside two or three other women who were taking his challenge to lose weight.

Source: JorgeCruise.com, Inc.

"I watched several other people diet and give up favorite foods like bread and meat and fats, you name it. I wanted a balance of all of these things because I knew after taking the dieting plunge so many times that I did not want to deprive myself or I would quit almost immediately as I always did. I knew that by the time I turned 40 I wanted to be at my goal weight of 150 pounds. I wanted to feel more energy and alive than I had ever felt and I wanted to do this for my family as well.

"I started eating the way Jorge recommended to us. Looking at my dinner plate in a whole new way seemed too easy but I loved it! It was unbelievable that first week I was feeling better than I had ever felt in years and I had lost 7 pounds!

"On my birthday I reached my goal weight and I felt younger and better than I ever have."

Michele's Secrets to Success

➤ Prioritize everything that is important, either in your head or on a calendar or piece of paper.

➤ Get ready the night before for your next day. Have lunches and dinners decided for the week so that when you go shopping you only get the things you need.

and not see results. Keep your salt intake below 2,000 milligrams a day. Switch from salt to a salt substitute such as Mrs. Dash® and read food labels. Many processed foods—particularly lunch meats and canned soups—are packed with salt. Try to eat more whole foods—fresh fruits and vegetables, whole-grain breads, and fresh fish and meat—and fewer processed and fast foods to lower your salt intake.

You've been exercising. If you've been incorporating my 8 Minute Moves® into your program, you've added some lean muscle, which may boost your weight on the scale. This is good weight, so don't stop! My 8 Minute Moves® will add about one quarter-pound of muscle per week, or about 1 pound per month. As I've mentioned before, this muscle will help rev up your metabolism and burn off more fat. Muscle is also more compact than fat, so even though adding muscle may cause your weight loss on the scale to stagnate, you'll probably notice that your measurements are still shrinking.

You're using the scale inappropriately. Your body weight fluctuates throughout the day and week, which is why I recommend you weigh yourself just once a week at the same time of day. You'll find, for example, that you weigh more later in the day than in the morning. This doesn't mean you've put on fat during the course of the day. It only means you have food in your tummy (which adds weight to the scale) and more fluids in your body (which also adds weight on the scale).

Also, different scales are calibrated differently. You may find that you weigh more on a friend's scale or the doctor's office scale than you do at home. Don't let this faze you. Stay on track by weighing yourself once a week, at the same time of day, on the same scale, wearing the same clothing, in the same location.

You weigh less than 150 pounds. In this case, you may need to switch to a slightly different eating plan. See page 258 for more about this.

If none of the above applies to you, you may be estimating your portion sizes incorrectly or be eating emotionally and not realizing it. For one week, write down everything you eat in a food diary as soon as you eat it. This will help keep you honest and help you uncover hidden sources of calories. Also, measure out all the foods you eat with measuring cups and spoons to make sure you are using the suggested portions in chapters 12 and 13.

Still Stuck?

Your body may have adjusted to your new way of eating or you may have reached a temporary set point. You can stimulate it to lose more weight, however, by exercising. Jump start your metabolism by adding lean muscle with the 8 Minute Moves® in chapter 11. If you are already doing 8 Minute Moves®, burn more calories each day by trying some power walking.

Have you reached your goal?

Congratulations! I'm so proud of you. To maintain your weight loss, you must continue the 3-hour lifestyle. I'd love to give you a one-size-fits-all blueprint that you can follow to maintain your success. Because not everyone's metabolism works quite the same way, however, you'll need to try the following experiment to find the best 3-hour maintenance option for you.

1. **Follow the same meal plan you've been following for one more week, and then weigh yourself on Sunday.** If you find you've lost another pound or two, double your snack size to 200 calories. You can easily do this by eating four snacks a day from the list of snacks in Chapter 12 rather than only two snacks a day. This will boost your daily calorie consumption to 1,650 calories. Then, move on to step 2. If, when you step on the scale, you are the same weight as the week before, continue with the 1,450-calorie plan. If your weight has decreased, go to step 2; if it increases, go to step 4.

2. **Follow your new meal plan for another week and then weigh yourself on Sunday.** If after one week at 1,650 calories a day you continue to lose weight, then raise your snacks to 300 calories each, for a total of 1,850 daily calories. If your weight is the same when you step on the scale, go to step 4.

3. **Follow this new meal plan for 1 week and then weigh yourself on Sunday.** If after one week at 1,850, you continue to lose weight, raise your snacks to 400 calories each for a total of 2,050 calories a day. If your weight is the same when you step on the scale, go to step 4.

4. **Stick with your new meal plan, weighing yourself each Sunday.** If you begin to gain weight, jump back to the previous week's calories selection. For example, if you are currently eating 2,050 calories a day but have recently gained a pound, jump back to eating only 1,650 calories a day.

Now, you've found your maintenance range. Over time you may need to adjust your maintenance plan depending on your lifestyle, your age, and how much you are exercising. So continue to weigh in each Sunday to stay on track.

Special Cases

Many people ask me whether it's safe for pregnant women and children to try the 3-Hour Diet.™. The answer to that question is yes and no. The 3-Hour Diet™ is a balanced way of eating. It's extremely healthy and good for growing children and pregnant women. That said, pregnancy and childhood generally are not times to be "dieting."

During pregnancy in particular, you are nurturing a growing baby. This baby needs plenty of protein, fat, and other nutrients for optimal brain and tissue development. Skimping on calories during this time will only jeopardize this important process. Pregnancy only lasts nine months. Promise me that you will wait until after you've birthed the baby to try to lose the weight!

If you breast-feed for one year, you will find that the weight comes off quite naturally. Many women find that they lose 10 pounds the day they deliver the baby and another 5 pounds in the next few weeks. After that, it takes about a year to lose the weight. So be patient. It will come off. Aim for a slow and steady 2- to 4-pound weight loss per month, especially if you are breast-feeding. Losing weight any faster may hinder your milk supply.

Following the 3-Hour Plate™ during pregnancy, however, can help make sure you consume the nutrients you need for a healthy baby. The plate will help you eat a balanced amount of protein, carbohydrates, and fats, along with a hefty dose of vegetables. These are all good for you and your baby. Just don't restrict yourself to small food portions. Eat when you feel hungry, even if that means adding in extra snacks, and continue to eat until you feel full. Let your body tell you when to eat and when to stop eating.

Just as the 3-Hour Plate™ can help pregnant women eat balanced, healthful meals, it also can help children do the same. Teach your children the power of the plate so they understand the importance of eating carbohydrates, proteins, and fats. This will teach them healthy habits that they can maintain for a lifetime.

A Special Program for Petite Women

If you are short in stature (5'3" or less) and weigh 150 pounds or less, you may plateau more quickly on the 3-Hour Diet™ than someone who has more weight to lose or is taller. A larger body burns more calories. That's all there is to it. As you lose weight, you'll need to adjust your diet accordingly.

So, if you weigh less than 150 pounds, the standard 3-Hour Diet™ may simple supply too much food. You can easily solve this issue by cutting your breakfast in half and eating only 200 calories during this meal. Continue to keep this meal balanced, consuming a mix of carbohydrates, proteins, and fats. Just eat half as much.

The Rest of Your Life

So there you have it, everything you need to stay on the 3-Hour Diet™ for life. Yep, make it a way of life—and a way of life you will love. Make the commitment today to become a "lifer" and you'll achieve long-lasting success.

BONUS EXERCISE OPTIONS

three years ago, I realized that I was looking at myself with blinders on. *I* didn't see the same person that the camera did. Since I started the 3-Hour Diet™ in March of 2004, I've learned a new lifestyle, complete with great support! Now, when I look in the mirror, I see a leaner body, minus three rolls. It amazes me to see how inches have melted away and it's fun to go shopping for clothes again!"

—BECKY GRAHN—LOST 40 POUNDS

This chapter is for those of you who also want to exercise while doing the 3-Hour Diet™. It will help give you an even more amazing body. The secret lies in my 8 Minute Moves®. With them, you'll be able to take the next step, further enhancing your shape and burning more calories to accelerate your results.

I encourage you to add 8 Minute Moves® to your program as soon as you feel you are able. I promise—they take only 8 minutes a day and they are the most enjoyable way to exercise.

Height: 5'7½"
Age: 33
Starting weight: 187 lbs.
Current weight: 135 lbs.
Other: a stay-at-home mom with 2 young children

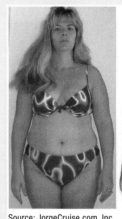

Source: JorgeCruise.com, Inc.

"Ten months ago, when I used to take the time to look in the mirror, I saw the following: Mother, Wife, Daughter, Sister, Niece, Granddaughter, Aunt, Cousin . . . the list goes on and on. I often put everyone and everything else first. At home I had a 2-month-old and a 3-year-old. I would do anything for them and decided a long time ago to be a stay-at-home mom. I think that is when I lost myself. I left behind any concern for my health and welfare when I had to start caring for others.

"I remember, before I got married, I started taking some diet pills that helped me to lose weight quickly. These pills were a quick, expensive fix, and a health risk as well. After my now 3-year-old son was born, I joined an expensive gym, wanting to make the effort. But of course I never went. I did not stick with either of these plans because of the lack of financial resources, lack of willpower, and feeling that being heavy was better than being sick from the pills.

"One New Year's Day I woke up. Something had to change in my life because I could not stand the person I had let myself become. The 3-Hour Diet™ changed my life. During the past nine months it has transformed more of me than I ever dreamed possible. Sure, I have lost most of the 52 pounds I set out to lose. Sure, I have transformed my body by doing great muscle toning exercise. I have changed my whole life by learning a wonderful, healthy way to live for the rest of my days!

"But along this journey something else happened. I have transformed myself on the inside as well. I love myself more. I love my husband and kids more (if that is possible). By looking out for ME first, I have been so much the better for it! When I look in the mirror now I have finally found ME behind the Mother, Wife, Daughter, and Sister."

Tasha's Secrets to Success

> ➤ Keep food temptations out of the house. When it's out of sight, it's out of your mouth.
> ➤ Plan your day and your week ahead of time.
> ➤ Always have healthy snacks in your car or purse so that you can stay on schedule.
> ➤ When you go to a social setting, try to focus on the importance of the people and not the food. Eat a healthy snack ahead of time or bring a healthy option to share.
> ➤ Stay focused on why you want to lose the weight and have a healthier lifestyle.

The 3-Hour Solution

My 8 Minute Moves® will help you to:

• Sculpt sexy shapes and curves
• Rebuild lost muscle that will further rev your metabolism and accelerate your results.

Why 8 Minutes of Strength Training?

These 8 minutes will help you to rebuild the lean muscle needed not only to burn fat faster, but also to sculpt and firm your shape. Although you can certainly shed weight through good nutrition alone, my 8 Minute Moves® will help you take your weight loss to the next level. They will help you create sexy contours to your arms and legs, firm and flatten your belly, and lift your tush.

Whereas your 3-Hour Diet™ plan will help you preserve the metabolism you now have, your 8 Minute Moves® will help you boost it to its highest possible level. It doesn't get any easier than this, folks.

The Beauty of 8 Minute Moves®

Unlike other strength-training programs, your optional 8 Minute Moves® sessions:

- Take only minutes a day to complete
- Require minimal equipment
- Can be done in your own home, even while wearing your PJs

How to Do the 8 Minute Moves®

In this chapter I have created two unique routines that will give you a great sample of the power of resistance training. I recommend that you complete one session on a Tuesday and another on a Thursday. This is the minimum amount of exercise you can do to stimulate muscle growth. If you want to accelerate your results even further, then make sure to check out my *8 Minutes in the Morning*® books or *Jorge's Cruise Control*™ videos at JorgeCruise.com.

Here's how the two special routines in this chapter work: On Tuesday you will work your upper body, and on Thursday your lower body. During each session, you will complete two moves. Do each of the two exercises for one minute each (about twelve repetitions). Repeat each exercise four times. Almost every single work out should last just 8 minutes. For example, on the day you work your upper body, you will do Knee Push-ups for 1 minute, followed by the Bird Dog for 1 minute. Then you will do Knee Push-ups again for 1 minute, and the Bird Dog again for 1 minute. You will continue alternating moves until your 8 minutes are up.

Here's how a typical Tuesday or Thursday morning should go for you:

- Warm up by jogging in place for 1 minute. The goal is to warm up your joints so that you avoid injury.
- Perform your 8 Minute Moves®.
- Cool down with the "Jorge Stretch." Sit on the floor with your left leg straight in front of you. Bend your right leg and put the sole of your right foot against the inside of your left thigh. Your legs will

Fifty and Fit

This 8 Minute Moves® model is one of my very own online clients, Nancy Bloom. She has lost an amazing 115 pounds and gone from a size 22 to a size 2 by eating every 3 hours and doing her 8 Minute Moves®. I am so proud of her success and her sculpted, slim body, that I wanted to showcase her here in this book.

Nancy's tip: Do exercises in the morning, before there are excuses not to do them later in the day.

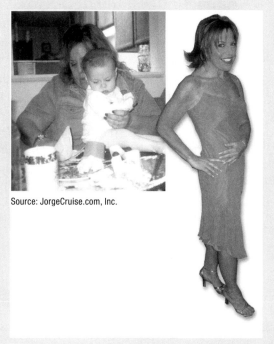

Source: JorgeCruise.com, Inc.

look like the number 4. With your left hand, try to touch either your left ankle or your left toe. This stretch works your left calf, Achilles tendon, hamstring, hip, knee, gluteus, lower-back muscles, shoulder, and wrist. Hold it for 30 seconds and then switch sides.

• Shower, change, and do whatever you need to do to face the day.
• Eat breakfast.

It's that easy. And remember, if these exercises become too simple or easy, we have a whole library of exercises in my *8 Minutes in the Morning*® books, Jorge's Cruise Control™ videos, and even on our online club.

Tuesday: Upper body

Chest

KNEE PUSH-UP Kneel on a mat on all fours with your knees hip-width apart, your hands slightly wider than shoulder-width apart, and your fingers pointing forward. Bring your pelvis forward so that your body creates a straight line from your knees to your head. Inhale as you lower your chest toward the floor, stopping once your elbows are even with your shoulders. Keep your back straight and your abdominals (stomach muscles) tight the entire time. Exhale as you push back up to the starting position, keeping your elbows slightly bent.

(Note: You can try doing wall push-ups if this exercise feels too hard.)

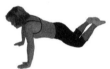 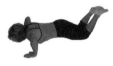

Back

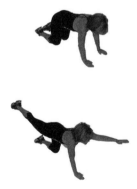

BIRD DOG Kneel on all fours on a mat. As you exhale, lift and extend your left arm and your right leg. Keep your back straight and abs tight throughout the move. When your arm and thigh are parallel to the floor, hold for a count of 3. Inhale as you lower them back to the starting position. Repeat with the opposite arm and leg. Continue to switch sides until you have completed your minute.

Thursday: Lower body

Quadriceps

SQUAT PUMP Stand with your feet directly under your hips. Extend your arms in front of you at shoulder height. Check your posture. Make sure your back is long and straight, your shoulders are relaxed away from your ears, and your abdomen is firm. As if you were going to sit back into a chair, inhale as you bend your knees and squat. Bend your knees no more than 90 degrees. (Only squat as deeply as you feel comfortable.) Make sure your knees remain over your ankles (not out past your toes). Keep your abdomen firm and your back straight as you squat. Exhale as you press up to the starting position. Repeat for 1 minute.

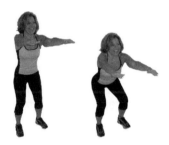

Hamstrings

LONG BRIDGE HOLD Lie on your back on an exercise mat or towel on the floor. Rest your arms at your sides and extend your legs, placing your heels against the seat of a chair (not pictured) or against the wall. Bend your knees slightly. Press into your heels as you exhale and lift your hips about 2 inches from the floor. Imagine you are a long bridge, like the Golden Gate Bridge in San Francisco. Hold for up to 60 seconds as you breathe normally.

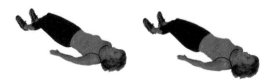

Power Walk Your Way to a Healthy Heart

Your 8 Minute Moves® are certainly your most convenient ticket to a faster metabolism and sculpted muscles, but you can do even more to accelerate your success. Some form of aerobic exercise, such as power walking, will not only help you burn off extra calories, but also will condition your heart and lungs, improving your overall health.

I'm a big fan of power walking. Each time you walk briskly for 20 minutes, you burn an additional 150 to 200 calories. If you walk 6 times a week during your lunch break, you'll burn an additional 1,200 calories. End result: power walking will help you meet your goal even faster.

I recommend you purchase a pedometer, a handy, inexpensive device sold at many sporting goods stores. Strap it to your waistband and keep track of how many steps you take in a typical day. Then, each day, try to walk more steps than you did the day before. Eventually, aim for 10,000 steps a day. That's the number researchers say will fully condition your heart and stimulate weight loss.

Although 10,000 steps may sound like a lot, you can easily add in more steps with the following tactics:

- Take a brisk 10-minute walk before work. It will help clear your mind and ready you for the day ahead.
- Walk to a coworker's office rather than send e-mail or call on the phone.
- Park in the spot farthest away from your destination. As an added bonus, this will help you save time because you no longer must circle the lot in search of one of the closest spaces!
- Drink plenty of water (which will boost your metabolism as well). You'll take more trips to the bathroom, increasing your walking time!
- Take mini–walk breaks throughout the work day. Even just 5 minutes around the building will help clear your mind and make you more productive.
- Walk with your family in the evening. It will bring you closer.

Exercise Equipment Made Easy

Now what if you want to use a gym or want to create your own home gym? What should you use? What are the essential pieces of equipment to a great gym? Well, the following are items I personally use and would recommend to you:

STRENGTH TRAINING

Dumbbells are the magic wand that will restore your lost lean muscles and rev up that metabolism even higher. Yep, dumbbells are small, portable, and easy to use almost anywhere. My very first *8 Minutes in the Morning*® book used these exclusively. My favorite ones are the chrome dumbbells made by Ivanko. They start at 3 pounds and go all the way to 35 pounds. Perfect and compact for any home and available at most gyms too.

CARDIO

When you can't go out and do a power walk, there are two pieces of equipment I recommend for an excellent, safe cardiovascular workout: the Precor® treadmill or the elliptical cross trainer. The treadmill made by Precor® focuses on giving you a low-impact, intense aerobic workout. A great thing about this product is it has a feature that allows the machine to change its incline or establish a "varied stride." When the machine varies up, it focuses on your quadriceps and hamstrings, and when the machine varies down, it focuses on your calf muscles. I use it almost every day.

Precor® treadmills provide a consistent and extremely comfortable workout for your power-walking needs. Their treadmills have a chip that establishes an integrative footplant technique, allowing the machine to make small adjustments to its speed based on your individual pace. Regular treadmills function in a lateral motion and push you through the stride, often times putting your body through more stress. The Precor® treadmills slow down or stop when your heel is planted, providing a steady and comfortable stride. My wife, Heather, loves this one best!

STRETCHING

After any workout it's ideal to stretch and increase flexibility. One of my favorite tools to stretch with is the Stretch Trainer by Precor®. It's fantastic and helps improve flexibility for everyday activities.

Visit JorgeCruise.com for links to all these brands.

TWELVE

3-HOUR PLATE™ CUSTOM-MEAL FOOD LISTS

grew up thin, with my parents begging me to eat. Back then, I was a picky eater. By age 18, however, I began to really enjoy food. By the time I met my husband, I weighed 165 pounds, and often joked that the word "diet" really meant "try-it," because every dish I saw I wanted to "try it"! By our fifth anniversary I weighed 208 pounds. One day, I saw Jorge on television, and decided to try his 3 Hour Diet™. He inspired me to take control of my life and change my eating habits. Within five weeks on his plan, I lost 15 pounds! It had taken a year to gain those pounds, but just over a month to lose them!"

—CELESTE ROBERTS—LOST 31 POUNDS

My 3-Hour Plate™ provides the simplest method to support you in your goal of healthy eating. There's no time-consuming calorie counting or banning of foods. As long as you fill the top half of your plate with veggies the equivalent of three DVD cases and the bottom half with protein the equivalent of a deck of playing cards and carbohydrates the equivalent of a Rubik's Cube® along with 1 teaspoon of fat the equivalent of a water bottle cap, you will provide your body a well-balanced nutritional meal (see page 87).

Some Suggested Guidelines

The following food lists are to be used with your 28-Day Planner (Chapter 9). If you ever feel confused about how much food to place on your 3-Hour Plate™, consult my simple food lists below.

Carbohydrates
Approximate portion size is equivalent to a Rubik's Cube®.

Fill in a Carbohydrate line on your 3-Hour Timeline™ by choosing one of the items listed below. Higher-fat selections will require you to fill in the Fat line in addition to the complex Carbohydrate line. If you can't find a particular complex carbohydrate listed, you can fill the line with any ½ cup of cereal, grain, pasta, or starchy vegetable.

BREADS

Bagel (½ of a 2-ounce bagel)

Bialy (½)

Biscuit (2½-inch diameter (1) PLUS 1 Fat line

Bread (1 ounce or 1 slice)

Bread, cocktail rye (3 slices)

Bread, low-calorie (2 slices)

Cornbread, 1 by 2 inches PLUS 1 Fat line

English muffin (½)

Hamburger roll (½)

Nan (bread from India) (¼ of an 8 by 2-inch loaf)

Pancake, low-fat, 4-inch diameter (2)

Pita, 6-inch (½)

Roll, dinner (1 small)

Taco shell, 6-inch (2) PLUS 1 Fat line

Tortilla, corn, 6-inch (1)

Tortilla, flour, 7-inch (1)

Waffle, fat-free (1)

GRAIN CEREALS AND GRAINS

Amaranth (⅛ cup)

Barley, cooked (½ cup)

Basmati rice, cooked (⅓ cup)

Brown rice, cooked (⅓ cup)

Buckwheat (Kasha), cooked (½ cup)

Bulgur, cooked (½ cup)

Cereal, cold, sweetened (½ cup)

Cereal, cold, unsweetened (¾ cup)

Cereal, hot, cooked (½ cup)

Couscous, cooked (½ cup)

Granola, low-fat (½ cup)

Hominy grits, cooked (½ cup)

Jasmine rice, cooked (⅓ cup)

Quinoa (⅛ cup)

Uncle Sam Cereal® (½ cup)

Wheat germ (3 tablespoons)

Wheat berries (⅛ cup)

Wild rice, cooked (⅓ cup)

White rice, cooked (⅓ cup)

FLOUR

Breadcrumbs, dry (3 tablespoons)

Cornmeal, dry (2½ tablespoons)

Cornstarch (2 tablespoons)

Matzo meal (⅓ cup)

Tapioca, uncooked (2 tablespoons)

Whole-wheat flour, all-purpose flour (2½ tablespoons)

PASTA

All varieties cooked such as spaghetti, linguine, noodles, penne (½ cup)

Orzo (½ cup)

Israeli Couscous (½ cup)

STARCHY VEGETABLES

Corn (½ cup)

Corn on the cob (6-inch ear)

French fries (10) PLUS 1 Fat line

Green peas (½ cup)

Potato, baked (1 small)

Potato, instant, prepared (1 cup)

Potato, mashed (½ cup)

Pumpkin (½ cup)

Sweet potato (⅓ cup)

Winter squash, acorn or butternut (¾ cup)

Kabocha (1 cup)

Yucca root (cassava), boiled (½ cup)

CRACKERS

Breadsticks, 4-inch long (2)

Chips, tortilla or potato, baked (¾ ounce or 15 to 20 chips)

Graham crackers, 2½-inch squares (3)

Matzo (¾ ounce)

Melba toast (4 slices)

Oyster crackers (24)

Popcorn (3 cups)

Rice cakes, plain (2 cakes)

Saltine crackers (6)

Soda crackers (4)

Whole-wheat crackers (2 to 5)

Protein
Approximate portion size is equivalent to a deck of playing cards

Fill in the protein line on your 3-Hour Timeline™ by choosing any **three** of the items below. It can be three: 1-ounce servings of a meat or fish, or you can mix and match with eggs, cheese, etc. Higher-fat selections will require you to fill in the fat line in addition to the Protein line. Meat protein sources are based on cooked portions (raw meat will shrink when cooking; a 4-ounce raw chicken breast will shrink to 3 ounces when cooked).

BEANS

Black, cooked (½ cup)

Black-eyed peas, cooked (½ cup)

Cannellini beans, cooked (½ cup)

Chickpeas, cooked (½ cup)

Flageolet beans, cooked (⅓ cup)

Garbanzo beans, cooked (⅓ cup)

All About Eggs

HARD-BOILED EGGS

Fresh eggs may be hard to peel, so it is best to use eggs that have been stored seven to ten days.

Start eggs in cold water with ½ teaspoon salt and 1 tablespoon oil. Bring to full boil, reduce the heat and simmer the eggs for 12 minutes or cover the pan, turn off the heat, and wait 15 to 20 minutes. Immediately put eggs in cold water to stop cooking process. Crack the shells and run them under cold water again. The eggs should peel easily. Hard-cooked eggs will keep in the refrigerator four to five days if left unpeeled.

IS THE EGG FRESH?

To determine whether an egg is fresh or not, immerse it in a pan of cool, salted water. If it sinks then it's fresh. If it rises to the surface throw it away!

EGG SALAD

For a little zip, add a little hot sauce or Worcestershire sauce.

HARD-BOILED OR FRESH?

Spin an egg on its side: if it spins it is hard-boiled; the fresh eggs won't spin.

FOR SALADS

Instead of chopping or slicing eggs for a salad, try grating them on the coarse side of a regular grater.

SUBSTITUTES FOR ONE WHOLE EGG IN A RECIPE

Mix 1 tablespoon cornstarch with 3 tablespoons extra liquid (whatever liquid is called for in the recipe); or use 2 tablespoons oil plus 1 tablespoon water; or use 2 tablespoons liquid plus 2 tablespoons flour, ½ tablespoon shortening, and ½ teaspoon baking powder.

General Shelf Life for Common Items and Frozen Foods

Flour, unopened: Up to 12 months; opened: 6 to 8 months.

Whole-wheat flour, unopened: 1 month; opened: 6 to 8 months if refrigerated.

Sugar, unopened: 2 years. Sugars do not spoil but eventually may change flavor.

Brown sugar, unopened: 4 months.

Confectioners' sugar, unopened: 18 months.

Solid shortening, unopened: 8 months; opened: 3 months.

Cocoa, unopened: indefinitely; opened: 1 year.

Whole spices: 2 to 4 years, whether or not opened.

Ground spices: 2 to 3 years, whether or not opened.

Paprika, red pepper, and chili powder: 2 years when kept in refrigerator.

High-acid canned items such as fruit juice, tomato soup, and foods in vinegar, unopened: 12 to 18 months.

Baking soda, unopened: 18 months; opened: 6 months.

Baking powder, unopened: 6 months; opened: 3 months.

Cornstarch: 18 months, whether or not opened.

Dry pasta made without eggs, unopened: 2 years; opened: 1 year.

Dry egg noodles, unopened: 2 years; opened: 1 to 2 months.

Salad dressing, unopened: 10 to 12 months; opened: 3 months if refrigerated.

Low-acid canned items such as soup, meats, gravy, and vegetables, unopened: 2 to 5 years.

Honey: 1 year, whether or not opened.

Worcestershire sauce: 1 year, whether or not opened.

Coffee, ground, canned, unopened: 2 years; opened: 2 weeks, if refrigerated.

Coffee, instant, in jars or tins, unopened: 12 months; opened: 3 months.

Water, bottled, unopened: 1 to 2 years; opened: 3 months.

Pudding mixes, unopened: 1 year; opened: 4 months.

Jams, jellies, and preserves, unopened: 1 year; opened: 6 months if refrigerated.

Peanut butter, unopened: 6 to 9 months; opened: 2 to 3 months.

SHELF LIFE FOR FROZEN FOODS

Meats:

Roasts: Beef, 6 to 12 months; lamb and veal, 6 to 9 months; pork, 3 to 6 months.

Steaks and chops: Beef, 6 to 9 months; lamb and veal, 3 to 4 months; pork, 2 to 3 months.

Poultry: Whole chicken, 1 year; chicken parts, 9 months; whole duck and turkey, 6 months; turkey parts, 9 months.

Seafood: Fatty fish (perch, mackerel, salmon), 2 to 3 months; white fish (cod, haddock, sole), 6 months; king crab, 10 months; raw shrimp, 12 months.

Cooked poultry, fish and seafood: 3 months.

Other Frozen Foods:

Produce items last longer than meats, if packaged properly. Frozen vegetables should last 8 to 10 months, frozen fruits a full year.

If freezing vegetables, be sure to blanch them first (except for onions, peppers and herbs); blanching destroys the enzymes that would cause them to deteriorate even when frozen. Fresh fruits should not be blanched, but they fare better when coated lightly with granulated sugar or mixed with a light sugar syrup.

When freezing baked goods, remember that commercial baked goods last longer, across the board, than home-baked ones. Commercially prepared frosted cakes and baked cookies, for example, last 8 to 12 months; home-baked cakes and cookies, only 3 months. Similarly, commercial yeast breads keep 3 to 6 months; home-baked breads, 3 months.

Other foods: Fruit juice concentrates, 12 months; butter, 6 to 9 months; margarine, 12 months; ice cream and sherbet, 2 months; frozen packaged entrees, 3 to 4 months; soups and stews, 2 to 3 months; salted nuts, 6 to 8 months; unsalted nuts, 9 to 12 months.

More freezing tips:

➤ If possible, remove excess air from containers; fold down bags to squeeze out all the air you can. (Exposure to air promotes rancidity.)

➤ If planning to freeze soup, use less liquid, stop cooking 10 minutes before the soup is finished and omit any potatoes. Add cooked potatoes or raw pasta and more liquid while reheating the soup over very low heat.

➤ Know which foods do not freeze well. Among them: watery vegetables such as cabbage, greens, celery, and cucumbers; fruits with delicate textures such as mangoes, pears, and avocados; cream sauces and custards; cooked potatoes; and plain cooked rice.

➤ Remember that a full freezer runs most efficiently. Just be mindful of what you've filled it with.

Hummus (¼ cup) PLUS the Fat line

Kidney, cooked (½ cup)

Lentil (red, black, or green), cooked (½ cup)

Lima, cooked (½ cup)

Navy, cooked (½ cup)

Pinto, cooked (½ cup)

Refried, fat-added (⅓ cup) PLUS the Fat line

Refried, fat-free (⅓ cup)

Small white (navy), cooked (½ cup)

Split peas, cooked (½ cup)

White (cannellini), cooked (½ cup)

CHEESE (55 CALORIES OR LESS PER OUNCE)

American (1 ounce)

Blue cheese (1 ounce)

Brie (1 ounce)

Cheddar (1 ounce)

Colby (1 ounce)

Cottage, low-fat or fat-free (¼ cup)

Feta (1 ounce)

Fontina (1 ounce)

Goat, part-skim (1 ounce or ¼ cup)

Gouda (1 ounce)

Havarti (1 ounce)

Jarslberg (1 ounce)

Monterey Jack (1 ounce)

Mozzarella, part-skim (1 ounce)

Muenster (1 ounce)

Neufchâtel, part-skim (1 ounce)

Parmesan, grated (1 tablespoon)

Provolone (1 ounce)

Ricotta, low-fat or fat-free (¼ cup)

Soy, all varieties (1 ounce)

Swiss (1 ounce)

MILK PRODUCTS

Buttermilk, low-fat or fat-free (¼ cup)

Evaporated skim milk (½ cup)

Lactose-free milk, low-fat or fat-free (6 ounces)

Milk, 1% or fat-free (6 ounces)

Nonfat dry (powder or reconstituted) milk
(¼ cup)

Rice milk, fortified, 1% or fat-free (6 ounces)

Soy milk, fortified, 1% or fat-free (6 ounces)

Yogurt, frozen, low-fat or nonfat (½ cup)

Yogurt, low-fat or nonfat, flavored, sweetened
with aspartame (6 ounces)

Yogurt, low-fat or nonfat, plain (6 ounces)

EGGS

Egg, whole (1)

Egg substitute (¼ cup)

Egg whites (3)

POULTRY

Chicken or turkey, white meat without skin
(1 ounce)

Duck, breast meat without skin (1 ounce)

Cornish Game Hen (1 ounce)

Goose, breast meat without skin (1 ounce)

Hot dog, turkey or chicken, reduced-fat or fat-
free (1)

FISH, CANNED

Salmon, packed in water (¼ cup)

Sardines, packed in water (2 medium)

White tuna, packed in water (¼ cup)

Freeze Tomatoes

Wash and core tomatoes (skin and seed if you care to). Place into freezer containers and freeze. They should last up to 1 year. You can use them as you would canned tomatoes.

FISH, FRESH OR FROZEN

Bluefish (1 ounce)	Monkfish (1 ounce)
Catfish (1 ounce)	Ono (1 ounce)
Calamari (1 ounce)	Orange roughy (1 ounce)
Cod (1 ounce)	Salmon (1 ounce)
Flounder (1 ounce)	Sea bass (1 ounce)
Fried fish (1 ounce) PLUS the Fat line	Shark (1 ounce)
Gefilte (2 ounces)	Snapper (1 ounce)
Grouper (1 ounce)	Sole (1 ounce)
Haddock (1 ounce)	Swordfish (1 ounce)
Halibut (1 ounce)	Trout (1 ounce)
Mackerel (1 ounce)	Tuna (1 ounce)
Mahimahi (1 ounce)	Yellowtail (1 ounce)

SHELLFISH

Clams (1 ounce)	Mussels (1 ounce)
Crab (1 ounce)	Oysters (6 medium)
Crawfish (1 ounce)	Scallops (1 ounce)
Lobster (1 ounce)	Shrimp (1 ounce)

When purchasing shellfish with the shells on, remember that the shells are part of the weight so take the shells into consideration. The portions listed above are out-of-the-shell, meat portions only.

SOY PRODUCTS

Soybeans, cooked (½)	Soy milk, fortified, 1% or fat-free (¾ cup ounces)
Soy burger (½ burger)	
Soy cheese (1 ounce)	Texturized soy protein (2 tablespoons or 1 ounce)
Soy hot dog (1)	
	Tofu (½ cup)

Freeze Peppers

Seed the peppers, put them in a freeze-lock plastic container, and freeze. Be aware that they will be slightly mushy but still good for sauces and such. (You can also freeze the peppers whole, this will result in a hotter pepper because of the seeds remaining intact.)

RED MEATS

Bacon, lean (1 slice)

Brisket (1 ounce)

Buffalo (1 ounce)

Goat (1 ounce)

Ground beef, pork, veal or combination
(1 ounce)

Ham, smoked or fresh (1 ounce)

Hot dog, beef, pork or combination, reduced-
fat or fat-free (1)

Lamb shank or shoulder (1 ounce)

Lamb loin, chop (1 ounce)

London broil (1 ounce)

Pork, chops, cutlets, shoulder or tenderloin
(1 ounce)

Pot roast (1 ounce)

Rib roast (1 ounce)

Round steak (1 ounce)

Sirloin steak (1 ounce)

Skirt steak (1 ounce)

Tenderloin (1 ounce)

Veal chop or roast (1 ounce)

Venison (1 ounce)

Fats
Approximate portion size is equivalent to a water bottle cap.

Fill in a Fat line on your 3-Hour Timeline™ by choosing one of the items below. Some fats are also considered protein and will take up both categories on your 28-day planner.

PREFERRED FATS

Almond butter (1 tablespoon) PLUS the Protein
line

Almonds, raw (6)

Avocado (⅛ medium)

Brazil Nut (2)

Canola oil (1 teaspoon)

Cashews (6)

Corn oil (1 teaspoon)

Flax oil (1 teaspoon or 4 capsules)

Oil-based salad dressing (1 tablespoon)

Olive oil (1 teaspoon)

Olives (10 small or 5 large)

Peanut butter (2 teaspoons) PLUS the Protein
line

Peanut oil (1 teaspoon)

Peanuts (10)

Pecans (4 halves)

Pesto sauce (1 tablespoon)

Pine nuts (1 tablespoon)

Pistachio nuts (1 tablespoon)

Pumpkin seeds (1 tablespoon)

Sesame seeds (1 tablespoon)

Soy mayonnaise (1 tablespoon)

Soy nuts (1 tablespoon)

Soy oil (1 teaspoon)

Sunflower seeds (1 tablespoon)

Tahini paste (2 teaspoons)

Walnuts (4 pieces)

FATS TO MINIMIZE

Alfredo sauce (1 tablespoon)

Bacon (1 slice)

Butter, reduced-calorie (1 tablespoon)

Butter, stick, (1 teaspoon)

Butter, whipped (2 teaspoons)

Coconut (2 tablespoons)

Cream cheese (1 tablespoon)

Cream cheese, reduced-calorie
 (2 tablespoons)

Gravy (½ cup)

Half-and-half (2 tablespoons)

Mayonnaise (1 teaspoon)

Mayonnaise, reduced-calorie (1 tablespoon)

Shortening (1 teaspoon)

Sour cream (2 tablespoons)

Sour cream, reduced-calorie (3 tablespoons)

Tartar sauce (1 tablespoon)

Vegetables and fruit
Approximate portion size is equivalent to 3 DVD cases.

VEGETABLES Vegetables that are high in starch do not appear on this list; they are on the carbohydrates list. Fill in the Veggie line on your Cruise Timeline™ by choosing one of the items below. All servings are 2 cups raw or 1 cup cooked, unless otherwise stated:

Artichoke, medium

Artichoke hearts, cooked

Asparagus

Bean Sprouts

Beet greens

Beets

Bell peppers (green, yellow, red)

Bitter Melon (Karela)

Broccoli

Brussels sprouts

Carrots

Cauliflower

Celeriac

Chard, Swiss

Chayote (squash)

Collard greens

Eggplant

Fennel bulb

Green beans

Kale

Kohlrabi

Leeks

Mung bean sprouts

Okra

Onions (1 cup raw, ⅔ cup cooked)

Parsnips

Pea pods

Pickles (4 large)

Pimento, sweet (1 cup)

Rutabaga

Sauerkraut

Scallion

Seaweed, raw

Snow peas

Spinach

String beans

Tomatillo, raw (2 medium)

Tomato (2 medium)

Tomato paste (4 tablespoons)

Tomato puree (1 cup)

Tomato sauce (1 cup)

Tomatoes, canned (1 cup)

Turnips

Vegetable juice, low sodium (1 cup)

Vegetable soup, fat-free, low sodium (1 cup)

FRUIT Fill in the Fruit line on your Cruise Timeline™ by choosing one of the items below. For fruits not listed, complete the Fruit line for every small to medium fresh fruit, ½ cup of canned fruit, or ¼ cup dried fruit. Ideally only eat fruit for breakfast due to higher simple sugar content.

Apples, green or red (1 medium)

Apple juice (½ cup)

Applesauce, unsweetened (½ cup)

Apricots, fresh (4)

Bananas (½ medium)

Blackberries (¾ cup)

Blueberries (¾ cup)

Boysenberries (¾ cup)

Cantaloupe (⅓ melon, or 1 cup cubes)

Casaba Melon (⅓ melon, or 1 cup cubes)

Cherries (12 large)

Clementine

Craisins (2 tablespoons)

Cranberries, unsweetened (1 cup)

Cranberry juice (½ cup)

Dates (3)

Figs, dried (1)

Figs, fresh (2)

Fruit cocktail (½ cup)

Grapefruit (½)

Grapefruit juice (½ cup)

Grapes, green or red (12)

Guava (1½ small)

Honeydew (⅛ melon, or 1 cup cubes)

Kiwifruit (1 large)

Mandarin orange sections (¾ cup)

Mango (½ medium)

Nectarine (1 medium)

Orange (1 medium)

Orange juice (½ cup)

Papaya (½ medium or 1 cup cubes)

Peach (1 medium)

Pear, green (1 small)

Pepino melon (1 cup cubes)

Persimmon (2)

Pineapple, canned and packed in juice, or
 fresh (⅓ cup)

Pineapple juice (½ cup)

Plum (2 medium)

Pomegranate (Chinese Apple) (½ medium)

Prickly pear (1 medium)

Prunes/dried plums (2)

Prune juice (⅓ cup)

Raisins (2 tablespoons)

Rhubarb, sweetened (½ cup)

Raspberries (1 cup)

Strawberries (1 cup)

Tangerine (2 small)

Watermelon (1 cup cubes)

Freebies

Freebies are foods that have less than 20 calorie: per serving. Some of these foods are limited since they can add up. Most of the following items do not need to be counted and can be consumed as often as you like. These are great items to use if you want a second plate of food or more than your two daily snacks. Enjoy them!

LIMITED

A1™ sauce (1 tablespoon)
Candy, hard, sugar-free (1)
Cocktail sauce (1 tablespoon)
Cocoa powder, unsweetened (1 tablespoon)
Cream cheese, fat-free (1 tablespoon)
Creamers, nondairy, liquid (1 tablespoon)
Creamers, nondairy, powdered (2 teaspoons)
Jam or jelly, low-sugar (2 teaspoons)
Margarine, fat-free (4 tablespoons)
Margarine, reduced-fat (1 teaspoon)
Mayonnaise, fat-free (1 tablespoon)
Mayonnaise, reduced-fat (1 teaspoon)
Onions (¼ cup)

Pickles (1½)
Relish, sweet pickle (1 tablespoon)
Salad dressing, fat-free (1 tablespoon)
Salsa (¼ cup)
Sour cream, fat-free or reduced-fat (1 tablespoon)
Soy sauce, light (2 tablespoons)
Syrup, sugar-free (2 tablespoons)
Taco sauce (1 tablespoon)
Teriyaki sauce (1 tablespoon)
Whipped topping, fat-free (2 tablespoons)
Worcestershire sauce (1 tablespoon)

VEGETABLES

Alfalfa sprouts
Cabbage
Celery
Cucumber
Green onions (scallions)
Jalapeño and other hot peppers

Jicama
Lettuce, all types (iceberg, loose leaf, romaine, spinach, watercress)
Mushrooms
Radishes
Zucchini

DRINKS

Canarino Italian hot lemon drink (canarino.com)
Carbonated or mineral water (add lime or lemon for great taste!)

Coffee, plain
Soft drinks, calorie-free
Tea

SPECIAL NOTE: For each beverage you drink that contains caffeine you must increase your water intake by 2 extra glasses to stay hydrated.

SEASONINGS

Chef Bernard's Fennel Pollen Spice Blends™ (www.chefbernard.com)

Garlic

Ginger

Herbs, fresh or dried

Kernel Season's Gourmet Popcorn Seasoning (kernelseasons.com—also excellent on pasta, vegetables, chicken, potatoes, eggs, and pitas)

Lawry's® Seasoned Salt

Lemongrass

Lemon pepper

Mrs. Dash®

Natural extracts (Lemon, Orange, Vanilla, Mint, etc.)

Nonstick olive oil cooking spray

Peppers and peppercorns (hot chile, black, white, pink, green)

Poppy seeds

Saffron

Salt (kosher, sea salt, fleur de sel, seasoning, Morton's)

Sesame seeds, pumpkin seeds (pepitas)

Spice blends (Cajun, curry, five spice, jerk, pickling, poultry)

Tabasco, hot pepper sauce

Togarashi (Japanese chili pepper)

Vanilla (whole bean, powder, paste, natural extract)

Wasabi powder

Star anise

CONDIMENTS

Cured Olives

Grape Seed Oil

Horseradish

Lemon juice

Lemon Myrtle Oil

Lime juice

Mustard

Nut oils (walnut, pistachio, almond, macadamia, hazelnut)

Pepperocinis

Pickled ginger

Pickle relish

Pickles, capers, cornichons

Salsa fresca

Sambal chili paste

Truffle oil

Vinegars (balsamic, seasoned Rice, sherry, naturally flavored)

Walden Farms Calorie-free salad dressings (waldenfarms.com)

Yuzu juice

SUGAR SUBSTITUTES

Equal®

Splenda® (splenda.com)

Sweet 'N Low®

SweetLeaf stevia products (steviaplus.com)- JORGE'S FAVORITE

MISCELLANEOUS

Chewing gum sugar-free

Gelatin sugar-free

Miscellaneous foods

For each of the foods on this list, the serving size is listed. You can substitute foods from this list for another food with the same number of calories. However, these foods do not contain as many important nutrients as the choices in the other sections. Since many of these foods are concentrated sources of sugar and calories, the portion sizes are often very small.

A1™ Sauce (2 tablespoons = 30 calories)
Barbecue sauce (2 tablespoons = 40 calories)
Chili sauce (2 tablespoons = 30 calories)
Chocolate syrup, light (2 tablespoons = 50 calories)
Cocktail sauce (¼ cup)
Fruit spread, 100% fruit (1 tablespoon = 54 calories)
Honey (1 tablespoon = 64 calories)
Hoisin sauce (2 teaspoons = 30 calories)
Ketchup (2 tablespoons = 30 calories)
Mole sauce (2 teaspoons = 75 calories)
Pancake syrup, reduced-calorie (2 tablespoons = 49 calories)
Soy Sauce (2 tablespoons = 20 calories)
Sugar, brown, light or dark (1 tablespoon = 33 calories)
Sugar, white, granulated (1 teaspoon = 15 calories; 1 tablespoon = 45 calories)
Sugar, white, powdered (1 tablespoon = 25 calories)
Syrup, maple (1 tablespoon = 52 calories)
Tamari, low-sodium (2 tablespoons = 20 calories)
Worcestershire sauce (2 tablespoons = 30 calories)

Alcohol

For maximum weight loss, alcohol should be kept to a minimum and limited to only special occasions. Fill in one Snack line for each of the specified amounts.

Beer (12 ounces)   Liquor (1½ ounces)
Beer, light (12 ounces)   Wine (5 ounces)

MEASUREMENT EQUIVALENTS

Dash or pinch	=	⅛ teaspoon or less
1 teaspoon	=	⅓ tablespoon
3 teaspoons	=	1 tablespoon
2 tablespoons	=	⅛ cup or 1 fluid ounce
4 tablespoons	=	¼ cup or 2 fluid ounces
5⅓ tablespoons	=	⅓ cup
8 tablespoons	=	½ cup or 4 fluid ounces
16 tablespoons	=	1 cup or 8 fluid ounces or ½ pint
⅓ cup	=	5 tablespoons + 1 teaspoon
⅞ cup	=	¾ cup + 2 tablespoons
2 cups	=	1 pint or 16 fluid ounces
4 cups	=	2 pints or 1 quart or 32 fluid ounces
4 quarts	=	8 pints or 1 gallon or 16 cups
1 pound	=	16 ounces
1 gram	=	a paper clip
1 gram	=	a dime
10 teaspoons	=	40 grams
1 ounce	=	28 grams or 0.125 cup or 29.57 milliliters
1 pound	=	16 ounces
8 ounces	=	236.6 milliliters

THIRTEEN

PREMADE-MEAL IDEAS

Before starting Jorge's program, I used to think,
"Damn, am I that fat?" whenever I looked in the
mirror. I just didn't feel as fat as I looked. When I
heard Jorge speak about his 3-Hour Diet™, it was
as if a lightning bolt struck me. His plan just made
sense. I have lost 10 pounds over the first month
of following Jorge's 3-hour plan. I have not been
hungry and have not had to work hard at it. I still
have a long way to go, but there is a light at the
end of the fat man tunnel."

—TOM BROWN—LOST 15 POUNDS

It is recommended that you purchase a weight scale for measurements of
certain homemade meal ingredients.

CONTENTS

Breakfast: Homemade

BACON AND POTATO OMELET

SERVES 4

Cooking spray	10 fresh spinach leaves, stems removed, sliced into ¼-inch ribbons
4 slices low-fat or turkey bacon, cut into small pieces	8 whole eggs, beaten slightly
¼ cup thinly sliced red onion	⅓ cup low-fat unflavored yogurt
3 small potatoes, peeled and sliced (¼ inch thick)	Salt and pepper
2 sprigs fresh thyme, leaves only, chopped	

Lightly spray a medium nonstick skillet with cooking spray. Add the bacon and onion, and cook over medium heat until lightly colored. Add the potatoes and thyme, and cook about 3–5 minutes, until bacon is crisp, onion is soft, and potatoes are browned. Remove from heat and add the spinach; gently mix. Transfer the mixture to a medium bowl.

Combine the eggs and yogurt in another bowl; season with salt and pepper. Pour into the same skillet. Spoon the bacon mixture evenly over the eggs. Cook over low heat without stirring. Lift the edges of the omelet and tilt the pan occasionally so the uncooked egg can run underneath and cook.

When the omelet is set on top, about 2–3 minutes, fold onto a serving plate and cut into 4 portions. Serve immediately.

Serve with ½ grapefruit each, or another fruit of your choice.

SAUSAGE AND CHEESE BREAKFAST BURRITO

SERVES 4

6 egg whites, lightly beaten	¼ cup drained roasted red pepper strips
2 whole eggs, lightly beaten	1 tablespoon chopped parsley
Salt and pepper	4 ounces grated low-fat cheese of your choice (about 1 cup)
Cooking spray	
4 ounces lean sausage, crumbled, cooked, and drained	4 (6-inch) tortillas, preferably whole-wheat

Combine the eggs and egg whites in a small bowl, and season with salt and pepper. Lightly coat a medium nonstick skillet with cooking spray. Add the eggs and cook over medium-low heat, stirring occasionally to scramble. When the eggs are almost set, sprinkle evenly with the sausage, red pepper, parsley, and cheese. Stir the mixture gently, and cook until the eggs are just set. Do not overcook.

Warm the tortillas in the microwave for 20 seconds on HIGH. Spoon one-quarter of the egg mixture onto each tortilla and roll into a burrito shape.

Serve with chilled cantaloupe and strawberries: Cut a cantaloupe into quarters and remove the seeds. Top each piece with ¼ cup of sliced fresh strawberries.

EGGS ON A CLOUD

SERVES 4

4 eggs, separated	4 (1-ounce) slices lean ham
Pinch of grated nutmeg	Salt and pepper
4 slices whole-wheat bread	4 ounces grated Swiss cheese (about 1 cup)
4 teaspoons butter	

Preheat the broiler.

Add a pinch of nutmeg to the egg whites and beat until stiff. Set aside.

Toast the bread lightly; spread each slice with 1 teaspoon of butter. Top each piece of toast with a slice of ham. Spoon the beaten egg whites on top of the ham. With the back of a spoon, make a slight indentation in the center of the egg whites and gently drop in an egg yolk. Season with salt and pepper. Sprinkle evenly with the cheese. Cook under the broiler for 2–3 minutes, until the egg yolks are set. Place immediately on serving plates.

Serve with mixed berries: In a small bowl, combine ½ cup each of fresh blackberries, blueberries, and raspberries. Divide the berries among the serving plates.

MEXICAN SCRAMBLED EGGS

SERVES 4

4 whole eggs	2 teaspoons butter
6 egg whites	6 ounces cooked ham, cut into strips
2 tablespoons water or nonfat milk	2 tablespoons diced green bell pepper
Salt and pepper	2 tablespoons diced green onion (scallions)
1 large tomato, peeled, seeded, and diced	4 (6-inch) tortillas, preferably whole-wheat
1 tablespoon chopped parsley	Salsa Topping (recipe follows)

Beat the eggs and egg whites with the water. Season with salt and pepper. Stir in the tomato and parsley, and set aside.

Melt the butter in a large nonstick skillet over low heat. Add the ham, green pepper, and onion, and sauté for 2 minutes. Pour in the eggs and cook, stirring occasionally, until set.

While the eggs are cooking, heat the tortillas in the microwave on HIGH for 20 seconds.

Divide the eggs onto 4 plates. Serve with the tortillas and Salsa Topping.

Salsa Topping

4 ripe red tomatoes, seeded and diced	1 teaspoon grated lemon or lime zest
⅓ cup thinly sliced red onion	½ hot red or green chile, seeds removed, minced
2 cloves garlic, crushed	
2 tablespoons chopped fresh cilantro	Salt and pepper
2 tablespoons lemon or lime juice	

Combine all ingredients in a medium bowl. Keep refrigerated until ready to use.

Monte Cristo Breakfast Sandwich

SERVES 4

8 slices low-calorie whole-wheat bread	⅓ cup 1% milk
4 ounces sliced cooked turkey breast	¼ teaspoon ground cinnamon
4 ounces sliced low-calorie Swiss cheese	Salt and pepper
4 whole eggs	4 teaspoons olive oil

Cover 4 slices of bread with the turkey and cheese, top with remaining bread.

Whisk together the eggs, milk, cinnamon, and salt and pepper in a shallow bowl. Carefully dip each sandwich in the egg mixture to coat both sides. Set aside each sandwich when dipped.

Heat the oil in a large nonstick skillet over medium-high heat. Cook the sandwiches about 3 minutes on each side, until the cheese has melted and the outside is lightly browned.

Serve with sautéed apple slices.

Stuffed Potato with Corn Salsa

SERVES 4

4 small baking potatoes, scrubbed well	4 ounces grated cheese of your choice (about 1 cup)
Cooking spray	
4 whole eggs, lightly beaten	4 tablespoons low-fat sour cream
4 slices low-fat bacon, cooked, drained, and crumbled	Pinch of paprika
	Corn Salsa (recipe follows)

Prick the potatoes with a fork and bake in a toaster oven at 375° or in a regular oven at 400° for 45 minutes to 1 hour, or cook in the microwave on HIGH for 20 minutes. Cut in half lengthwise. Scoop out the pulp, chop lightly, and set aside; keep the skins warm.

Spray a medium nonstick skillet with cooking spray. Add the eggs and cook over low heat, stirring occasionally. When almost set, add the potato pulp and bacon. Cook until set.

INGREDIENT SUBSTITUTIONS

1 teaspoon baking powder	= ½ teaspoon cream of tartar + ¼ teaspoon baking soda
1 cup buttermilk	= 1 tablespoon lemon juice or vinegar + milk to make 1 cup
1 cup cake flour	= 1 cup – 2 tablespoons all-purpose flour
1 cup light brown sugar	= ½ cup packed brown sugar + ½ cup granulated sugar
1 cup powdered sugar	= ½ cup + 1 tablespoon granulated sugar
1 square (1 ounce) semisweet chocolate	= ½ square (½ ounce) unsweetened chocolate + 1 tablespoon sugar
1 square (1 ounce) unsweetened chocolate	= 3 tablespoons unsweetened cocoa + 1 tablespoon shortening or vegetable oil
1 tablespoon cornstarch	= 2 tablespoons all-purpose flour
1 cup light corn syrup	= 1¼ cups granulated sugar + ¼ cup liquid (whatever the recipe calls for)
1 cup cracker crumbs	= 1 cup dry bread crumbs
1 cup half-and-half (for cooking and baking)	= 1½ tablespoons melted butter + whole milk to make 1 cup
1 medium clove garlic, minced	= ¼ teaspoon garlic powder
1 teaspoon garlic salt	= ⅛ teaspoon garlic powder + salt to make 1 teaspoon
1 cup honey	= 1¼ cups granulated sugar + ⅓ cup liquid (whatever the recipe calls for)
1 teaspoon lemon juice	= ½ teaspoon vinegar
1 teaspoon grated lemon zest	= ½ teaspoon lemon extract
½ small onion, chopped (¼ cup)	= 1½ teaspoons dried minced onion OR ¾ teaspoon onion powder
1 tablespoon prepared	= 1 teaspoon powdered mustard + ¼ teaspoon mustard vinegar (or other liquid)
1 cup sour cream	= 1 cup unflavored yogurt (do not boil)
2 teaspoons tapioca	= 1 tablespoon all-purpose flour
1 cup tomato juice	= ½ cup tomato sauce + ½ cup water
2 cups tomato sauce	= ¾ cup tomato paste (6-ounce can) + 1 cup water
1 cup whole milk	= ½ cup evaporated milk + ½ cup water

INGREDIENT SUBSTITUTIONS

1 packet Equal® or Sweet 'N Low®	= 2 teaspoons granulated sugar
1 whole egg (for thickening only)	= 1 tablespoon cornstarch + 3 tablespoons liquid (whatever the recipe calls for) OR 2 tablespoons oil + 1 tablespoon water OR 2 tablespoons liquid + 2 tablespoons all-purpose flour + 1½ teaspoons shortening + ½ teaspoon baking powder

TO SUBSTITUTE APPLESAUCE FOR SHORTENING

You can substitute applesauce for shortening one for one up to 1 cup. This means you can use 1 cup applesauce for 1 cup shortening. Beyond 1 cup, use oil or shortening for the remainder of the amount. So if your recipe called for 1½ cups shortening you would use 1 cup applesauce and ½ cup shortening.

Spoon the egg mixture into the potato skins and sprinkle with the cheese. Garnish with the sour cream, paprika, and Corn Salsa (recipe follows).

Serve each potato (2 halves) with 1 orange, cut into wedges.

Corn Salsa

½ cup cooked fresh or frozen corn kernels	1 tablespoon finely chopped green bell pepper
¾ cup seeded, diced fresh tomato (1 large tomato)	1 tablespoon minced fresh cilantro
¼ cup finely peeled, chopped cucumber	1 tablespoon fresh lemon juice
2 tablespoons thinly sliced green onions (scallions)	1 teaspoon finely chopped seeded jalapeño chile
1 teaspoon olive oil	Salt and pepper

Combine all ingredients in a medium bowl. Cover and set aside until ready to serve.

EGGS NEST FLORENTINE

SERVES 4

Salt	½ cup freshly grated Parmesan cheese (about 2 ounces)
2 pounds loose or 2 (10-ounce) bags fresh spinach	½ cup plain fresh bread crumbs
Cooking spray	Grated zest of 1 orange
Pepper	2 tablespoons slivered almonds
1 tablespoon butter or olive oil, or 1½ teaspoons of each	4 slices whole-wheat bread or 2 split whole-grain English muffins
8 whole eggs	

Bring a large pot of salted water to a boil, and fill a large bowl with ice and water. Preheat the oven to 350°.

Wash the spinach thoroughly and remove tough stems. Cook in the boiling water for 1 minute. Drain and shock in the ice water. Drain well when cold and squeeze out all moisture. Chop very coarsely.

Lightly coat a 9 by 13-inch baking dish with cooking spray. Melt the butter in a skillet over low heat; add the spinach, season with salt and pepper, and stir thoroughly. Spread the spinach evenly over the bottom of the baking dish.

With the back of a spoon, make indentations in the spinach to form 8 nests. Crack 1 egg into each indentation. Combine the cheese, bread crumbs, orange zest, and almonds. Sprinkle the mixture evenly over the eggs.

Bake about 12 minutes, until the egg whites are set. While the eggs are baking, toast the bread or English muffins and place 1 piece on each of 4 plates. Top the bread with 2 spinach-egg nests and serve.

SALMON BAGELS

SERVES 4

6 whole eggs	Cooking spray
1¾ cups (one 14-ounce can) reduced-sodium chicken broth	4 medium regular bagels, spilt
¼ cup thinly sliced green onions (scallions)	1 (3-ounce) package thinly sliced smoked salmon
2 cloves garlic, minced	4 ounces grated Jack cheese (about 1 cup)
1 tablespoon chopped fresh dill or ¾ teaspoon dried dill weed	

Preheat the oven to 350°.

Beat the eggs and broth in a medium mixing bowl. Add the onions, garlic, and dill.

Lightly coat a 2-quart baking dish with cooking spray. Arrange the bottom halves of the bagel in the dish, cut side up. (It's okay if they overlap a little.) Layer the salmon on top of the bagel pieces. Sprinkle with the cheese. Place the remaining bagel pieces on top, cut side down. Gradually pour the egg mixture over all. Press down lightly with a spatula to submerge the bagels.

Bake uncovered for 30 minutes, until set and a knife inserted in the center comes out clean. Let stand for 10 minutes before serving.

Garnish with a side of fruit.

RANCHERO EGGS

SERVES 4

Cooking spray	4 whole eggs
1 large onion, halved and thinly sliced	Salt and pepper
1 (15-ounce) can chunky chili-style tomato sauce	4 ounces grated Jack or Cheddar cheese (about 1 cup)
1 fresh jalapeño chile, seeded and finely chopped	4 whole-wheat tortillas (6 inch) or 4 slices whole-wheat bread
2 tablespoons fresh oregano, leaves only, chopped	

Preheat the oven to 400°. Lightly coat a medium ovenproof skillet with cooking spray. Heat the skillet over medium-high heat. Add the onion and cook until tender, about 3 minutes, stirring occasionally. Remove from the heat.

In a small bowl, mix the tomato sauce, jalapeño, and oregano. Pour the mixture over the onions [and stir]. One by one, break the eggs into a small cup and carefully slide onto the tomato sauce, so that each quarter of the skillet has 1 egg. Season with salt and pepper. Bake uncovered for 10 minutes, until the egg whites are almost set.

While the eggs are baking, warm the tortillas in the microwave for 20 seconds on HIGH or toast the bread. When the eggs are ready, sprinkle evenly with the cheese and bake for 1 minute more. Divide the eggs and sauce among 4 serving plates.

Serve with the tortillas and 1 portion of low-fat fruit-flavored yogurt.

Ham and Potato Scramble

SERVES 4

1 tablespoon butter	¼ cup thinly sliced green onions (scallions)
1 cup refrigerated shredded hash brown potatoes	2 tablespoons chopped fresh basil
	¼ teaspoon garlic salt
½ cup diced low-fat cooked ham	¼ teaspoon ground black pepper
6 whole eggs	¼ teaspoon generic chili pepper powder
2 tablespoons nonfat milk	3 ounces grated reduced-fat Cheddar cheese (about ¾ cup)
1 tablespoon water	

Melt the butter in a medium nonstick skillet over medium heat. Add the potatoes and ham and cook 6 to 8 minutes, stirring occasionally. While the potatoes and ham are cooking, lightly beat the eggs with the milk and water. Stir in the onions, basil, garlic salt, pepper, and chili powder.

When the potatoes are lightly browned, pour the egg mixture over the potatoes. Let it cook over without stirring until the bottom begins to set, about 1–2 minutes. Lift the edges with a spatula and tilt the pan so the uncooked eggs can flow underneath. Continue cooking for 2 to 3 minutes more, until the eggs are cooked through but still moist on top. Remove from the heat; sprinkle with the cheese. Cut into 4 portions.

Serve each portion with half a slice of whole-wheat toast and sliced straw-berries.

VEGETABLE FRITTATA

SERVES 4

Cooking spray	1 small zucchini, halved lengthwise and cut into ¼-inch slices (about ¾ cup)
1 tablespoon butter	
1½ pounds fresh asparagus, trimmed, peeled, and cut into 1-inch pieces	1 baby eggplant, cut into ¼-inch cubes (about ¾ cup)
1 medium yellow bell pepper, cut into ¼-inch strips	8 whole eggs
	1 cup low-fat milk
⅓ cup chopped onion	2 tablespoons chopped fresh basil
	Salt and pepper

Preheat the oven to 350°. Lightly coat a 2-quart casserole with cooking spray.

Melt the butter in a large skillet over medium heat. Add the asparagus, pepper, onion, zucchini, and eggplant, and sauté about 2–3 minutes, until the vegetables are crisp-tender. Spread the vegetables evenly in the casserole.

In a medium bowl, combine the eggs, milk and basil. Season with salt and pepper. Pour the egg mixture over the vegetables. Bake uncovered about 35 minutes, until a knife inserted in the center comes out clean. Let stand 10 minutes before serving.

Serve with a slice of toast.

GRANOLA WITH YOGURT

SERVES 4–6

Cooking spray	2½ cups regular rolled oats
⅓ cup unsweetened pineapple juice or apple juice	1 cup wheat flakes
	⅓ cup toasted wheat germ
⅓ cup honey	⅓ cup sliced almonds and chopped pecans, mixed (about fifty-fifty)
¼ teaspoon ground allspice	
¼ teaspoon ground cinnamon	

Preheat the oven to 325°. Lightly coat a shallow baking dish with cooking spray.

Combine the juice, honey, allspice, and cinnamon in a small saucepan. Place over medium heat and bring just to a boil; remove from the heat.

While the liquids are heating, combine the oats, wheat flakes, wheat germ, and nuts in a large bowl. Pour the liquid over; toss to coat thoroughly. Spread the mixture evenly in the baking dish.

Bake about 30 minutes, stirring 2 or 3 times, until the oats are lightly browned. Turn out onto a large piece of foil and let cool completely.

Store in a sealed container in the freezer for up to 3 months or in the refrigerator for up to 2 weeks.

For each serving, spoon 1 cup of unflavored low-fat yogurt into a bowl. Top with ½ cup of the granola and ½ cup mixed fresh fruit (blackberries, raspberries, blueberries, sliced strawberries, etc.).

Mock Danish

SERVES 4

2 cups diced pineapple (if using canned pineapple, drain well first)	1 teaspoon ground cinnamon
	4 packets (1 gram each) sugar substitute
1 cup cottage cheese	4 slices bread, preferably whole-grain
¼ teaspoon vanilla extract	

Preheat the broiler.

In a medium bowl, combine the pineapple, cottage cheese, vanilla, cinnamon, and sugar substitute. Toast the bread lightly on one side. Spread the topping mixture on the untoasted side, and place under the broiler until heated.

Add 2 soft-boiled eggs topped with 1 teaspoon of butter to each serving to complete the meal.

Breakfast: Frozen Meals

LEAN POCKETS® SAUSAGE, EGG AND CHEESE (1)
Add ½ cup of low-fat cottage cheese and your choice of fruit, either an apple or peach, or mix it up by having a cup of mixed berries.

EASY OMELETS® OMELET, CHEDDAR FLAVOR
Add one piece of fruit of your choice.

EGGO®: NUTRI-GRAIN LOW-FAT BLUEBERRY WAFFLES (2)
Add a fluffy mixture of 2 eggs (or 6 egg whites) scrambled with water and 1 ounce of the cheese of your choice. Top it off with a piece of fruit or a cup of berries and enjoy!

Note: When preparing eggs in a nonstick skillet, use cooking spray if necessary.

EGGO®: NUTRI-GRAIN LOW-FAT WAFFLES (2)
Spread 1 teaspoon of peanut butter on the waffles. Prepare 3 slices of lean turkey bacon and add a glass of 1% milk or ¼ cup of low-fat cottage cheese. Don't forget to add the fruit and have a delicious breakfast.

WEIGHTWATCHERS® SMART ONES® ENGLISH MUFFIN SANDWICH (1)
Add a medium piece of fruit or 1 cup of assorted berries.

AMY'S KITCHEN® APPLE OR STRAWBERRY & CREAM TOASTER POPS (1)
Add a piece of fruit or a couple eggs.

AMY'S KITCHEN® TOFU SCRAMBLE IN A POCKET SANDWICH
Add a piece of fruit.

Breakfast: Fast Food

These selections are the healthiest options that fall into the criteria of the Cruise Down Plate®.

McDONALD'S® EGG MCMUFFIN® (1)
Add 1 glass of 1% milk and a medium piece of fruit or a 1 cup assortment of mixed berries.

JACK IN THE BOX® BREAKFAST JACK®

Add 1 glass of 2% milk and a medium piece of fruit or 1 cup of berries for a great breakfast treat.

HARDEE'S® FRISCO® BREAKFAST SANDWICH

Add a medium piece of fruit or mix and match with a cup of assorted berries.

ARBY'S® SOURDOUGH, EGG 'N CHEESE SANDWICH

Add a medium piece of fruit or 1 cup of assorted berries.

NOTE: Visit JorgeCruise.com for the newest homemade, frozen, and fast-food ideas in our Success News section.

LUNCH/DINNER

CONTENTS

Lunch/Dinner: Homemade

ZUCCHINI QUICHE

SERVES 6

Cooking spray	1⅓ cup nonfat milk
2 teaspoons olive oil	3 egg whites
¾ pound zucchini, thinly sliced	1 whole egg
½ teaspoon Cajun spice mix	¾ cup low-fat buttermilk baking mix
5 ounces grated Swiss cheese (about 1¼ cups)	Salt and pepper
	2 medium tomatoes, cut into ⅛-inch slices

Preheat the oven to 375°. Lightly coat a 10-inch pie pan with cooking spray.

Heat the oil in a medium skillet over medium-high heat. Add the zucchini, season with the Cajun spices, and sauté for 3 to 4 minutes, stirring often, until just softened.

Place the zucchini in the pie pan in an even layer. Sprinkle with two-thirds of the cheese.

In a medium bowl, beat together the milk, egg whites, egg, and baking mix. Season with salt and pepper. Pour over the zucchini and cheese.

Bake uncovered for 25 to 35 minutes, until a knife inserted in the center comes out clean. Cover with the tomato slices, and sprinkle with the remaining cheese. Bake 1 to 2 minutes longer, until the cheese is lightly browned. Let stand for 5 minutes before cutting into 6 pieces.

To complete your meal add a tossed salad.

DELI PASTA SALAD

SERVES 4

1 (8- to 9-ounce) package frozen or refrigerated cheese-filled tortellini (about 2 cups)	1 teaspoon dried Italian seasoning
	1 teaspoon Dijon mustard
1½ cups broccoli florets	¼ teaspoon ground black pepper
¾ cup thinly sliced carrots	⅛ teaspoon garlic powder
¾ cup chopped yellow or red bell pepper	2 tablespoons minced fresh basil
1 tablespoon olive oil	2 heads Bibb or butter lettuce, separated, washed, and patted dry
1 tablespoon flax oil	1 cup low-fat cottage cheese
¼ cup white wine vinegar	4 hard-boiled eggs, peeled and sliced

Bring a large pot of water to a boil and cook the pasta according to the package directions. Two minutes before the end of the cooking time, add the broccoli, carrots, and bell pepper. The pasta should be cooked tender and the vegetables should be crisp-tender. Drain, rinse with cold water, and drain well. Transfer to a large mixing bowl.

Combine the oils, vinegar, Italian seasoning, mustard, black pepper, and garlic powder in a small screw-top jar and shake well. Pour the dressing over the pasta and vegetables, add the basil, and toss to coat well.

Arrange the lettuce leaves on 4 serving plates. Scoop one-quarter of the pasta salad onto part of the lettuce on each plate. Add ¼ cup of the cottage cheese and 1 sliced egg to each plate.

ARTICHOKE PITA

SERVES 4

1 (15-ounce) can black-eyed peas, rinsed and drained	½ cup low-fat creamy garlic salad dressing
	¼ teaspoon cracked black pepper
1 (14-ounce) can artichoke hearts, drained and cut into small pieces	2 (6-inch) whole-wheat pitas
	1 medium tomato, sliced thin
2 tablespoons chopped green onions (scallions)	1 small cucumber, peeled and sliced very thin
2 cups finely chopped mixed salad greens	

In a large bowl, mix the peas, artichokes, green onions, salad greens, salad dressing, and pepper. Cut the pitas in half to form 4 pockets and open. Line each pita pocket with slices of tomato and cucumber. Spoon one quarter of the artichoke mixture into each.

SHRIMP STIR-FRY SALAD WITH CORN AND BLACK BEANS

SERVES 4

2 teaspoons olive oil	1 teaspoon butter
1 cup fresh or thawed corn kernels	1 teaspoon sugar substitute
2½ tablespoons minced fresh ginger	¾ cup chopped green onions (scallions)
2 cloves garlic, minced	Salt and pepper
1 shallot, minced	1 bag "European" or other packaged salad mix
1½ pounds raw medium shrimp, peeled and deveined	
	2 tomatoes, cut into wedges
1 (15-ounce) can black beans, rinsed and drained	¼ cup chopped fresh cilantro
	2 tablespoons toasted chopped cashews

Heat the oil in a wok or large nonstick skillet over medium heat. Add the corn, ginger, garlic, and shallot and sauté for 2 minutes without browning. Add the shrimp and stir-fry for 2 minutes more. Add the beans, butter, and sugar substitute. Stir-fry for 3 minutes more, stirring frequently. Remove from the heat. Fold in the green onions. Season with salt and pepper.

Divide the salad greens among 4 serving plates. Spoon the shrimp mixture over the salad. Garnish with tomato wedges and sprinkle with the cilantro and cashews.

SALAD-STUFFED PITAS

SERVES 4

½ head iceberg lettuce, cut into fine strips	8 black olives, pitted and chopped
½ medium cucumber, peeled and diced	2 (6-inch) whole-wheat pitas
9 cherry tomatoes, halved	2 cups sunflower sprouts
½ cup finely chopped green onions (scallions)	Dressing (recipe follows)
½ cup crumbled feta cheese (about 2 ounces)	

In a large bowl, combine the lettuce, cucumber, tomatoes, onions, cheese, and olives. Add the dressing and toss well to mix.

Cut the pitas in half to form 4 pockets and open. Divide the salad into 4 portions and fill the pita halves. Garnish with the sprouts.

Enjoy with a light fruit-flavored yogurt on the side. (Yoplait Light® has only 100 calories.)

Dressing

1 clove garlic, minced	2 tablespoons olive oil
⅛ teaspoon salt	1 teaspoon chopped fresh mint
2 teaspoons lemon juice	⅛ teaspoon ground black pepper

Combine the dressing ingredients in a small screw-top jar. Cover and shake well. Set aside.

SANDWICH WRAP I

SERVES 4

4 (6-inch) whole-wheat tortillas or reduced-calorie tortillas	4 ounces shredded Jack cheese (about 1 cup)
Prepared mustard of your choice	1 cup chopped iceberg lettuce
4 tablespoons reduced-fat mayonnaise	½ cup diced tomatoes
8 ounces cooked ham, turkey, or roast beef (your choice of one), thinly sliced or cut into ¼-inch cubes	¼ cup minced green onion (scallion)

Spread each tortilla with mustard and mayonnaise. Layer each with one quarter of the meat, cheese, lettuce, tomato, and onion. Wrap tightly in a burrito shape.

Serve with 1 cup of fat-free vegetable soup or a salad.

SANDWICH WRAP II

SERVES 4

4 (6-inch) whole-wheat tortillas or reduced-calorie tortillas	½ avocado, sliced
Prepared mustard of your choice	1 small head butter or Bibb lettuce, cut into ½-inch strips
8 ounces cooked ham, turkey, or roast beef (your choice of one), thinly sliced or cut into ¼-inch cubes	½ cup diced tomatoes
	½ cup alfalfa sprouts
4 ounces smoked Cheddar cheese, sliced or shredded (about 1 cup shredded)	¼ cup thinly sliced red onion

Spread each tortilla with mustard. Layer each with one quarter of the meat, cheese, avocado, lettuce, tomato, sprouts, and onion. Wrap tightly in a burrito shape.

Serve with 1 cup of fat-free vegetable soup or a salad.

ITALIAN MOZZARELLA SALAD

SERVES 4

5 ounces baby spinach, washed and dried	2 tablespoons chopped fresh Italian (flat-leaf) parsley
4½ ounces watercress, washed and dried	2 teaspoons balsamic vinegar
3½ ounces mozzarella cheese, cut into small cubes	2 tablespoons extra virgin olive oil
7 ounces ham or salami, cut into strips	Salt and pepper
1 pint cherry tomatoes, cut in half	

Place the spinach and watercress in a large salad bowl. Add the mozzarella, ham, tomatoes, and parsley in order. Sprinkle with the vinegar and oil, season with salt and pepper, and toss to coat. Serve at once.

Tomato Stuffed with Tuna

SERVES 4

4 large tomatoes	Pinch of cayenne pepper
2 (3-ounce) cans water-pack tuna, drained	Salt and pepper
2 tablespoons reduced-fat mayonnaise	1 head red or green leaf lettuce, separated, washed, and patted dry
4 tablespoons chopped celery	
4 tablespoons chopped onion	4 hard-boiled eggs cut into slices
2 tablespoons lemon juice	

Cut the tops off the tomatoes and scoop out and discard the seeds and tops. Place the tomatoes upside down on paper towels to drain.

In a medium bowl, combine the tuna, mayonnaise, celery, onion, lemon juice, and cayenne. Season with salt and pepper.

Place 2 lettuce leaves on each of 4 serving plates and top with a tomato. Divide the tuna mixture among the tomatoes, and garnish with slices of hard-boiled egg.

Include a small dinner roll.

Pasta Salad

SERVES 4

2 cups cooked preferred pasta rinsed and drained (about 1¼ cups or 4 ounces uncooked)	1 pint cherry tomatoes, cut in half
	16 pitted black olives, sliced
1 cup broccoli florets, cooked and chilled	8 basil leaves, cut into thin strips
1 cup cauliflower florets, cooked and chilled	¼ cup low-fat Italian dressing

Gently toss together the pasta, broccoli, cauliflower, tomatoes, olives, basil, and dressing in a large salad bowl. Serve at once.

This pasta salad can accompany 6-ounce skewers of grilled garlic shrimp or 3-ounce herb-baked chicken breasts.

BEEF AND BROCCOLI STIR-FRY WITH APPLE-SESAME SALAD

SERVES 4

12 ounces trimmed lean steak	¼ cup beef broth
2 cloves garlic, crushed	Juice and grated zest of 1 orange
Dash of chili oil	2 teaspoons cornstarch
½-inch piece of ginger, grated	4 teaspoons water
½ teaspoon Chinese 5-spice powder	2 cups steamed rice (from ⅔ cup raw regular rice or 1 cup instant)
3 tablespoons soy sauce	
2 tablespoons olive oil	¼ cup thin carrot strips
½ pound broccoli florets	2 tablespoons chopped fresh cilantro

Cut the steak into thin strips and place it in a shallow bowl. Add the garlic, chili oil, ginger, Chinese 5-spice, and 2 tablespoons of the soy sauce. Stir to coat the meat. Cover the bowl and place in the refrigerator to marinate for at least 2 hours. While the meat is marinating, start the Apple-Sesame Salad (recipe follows).

Heat 1 tablespoon of the olive oil in a wok or large skillet over medium heat. Add the broccoli and stir-fry for 4 to 5 minutes. Remove with a slotted spoon and set aside. Add the remaining tablespoon of olive oil to the wok and heat medium high. Add the marinated steak and stir-fry for 2 to 3 minutes, until brown and seared. Return the broccoli to the wok, and add the remaining tablespoon of soy sauce, the orange juice, and the beef broth. Blend the cornstarch and water in a small bowl. Bring the mixture in the wok to a boil and add the cornstarch slurry, stirring until the sauce is thick and clear. Cook for 1 minute more.

Put ½ cup of rice on each serving plate and top with the meat, broccoli, and sauce. Garnish with carrot strips. Sprinkle with the orange zest and the cilantro. Serve with a side of Apple-Sesame Salad.

Apple-Sesame Salad

2 cups fresh bean sprouts	3 stalks celery, cut into 1-inch pieces
1½ tablespoons chopped fresh mint	1 large red bell pepper, cut into small pieces
3 tablespoons fresh lime juice	1 large Granny Smith apple, cored and cut into small chunks
½ teaspoon mild chili powder	
1 teaspoon sugar substitute	2 tablespoons toasted sesame seeds
½ teaspoon salt	

Soak the bean sprouts in ice water for 10–15 minutes; clean and drain. (They should be fresh and crunchy.) Place them in a large serving bowl and keep refrigerated.

For the dressing, combine the mint, lime juice, chili powder, sugar substitute, and salt in a small bowl and mix thoroughly. Set aside.

Add the celery, pepper, and apples to the bean sprouts and mix gently. Just before serving pour the dressing over the salad and toss well to mix. Sprinkle with the sesame seeds.

VEGETABLE ENCHILADAS

SERVES 4

Sauce

1¼ cups canned strained tomatoes	1¼ cups vegetable stock
1 shallot, chopped	1 teaspoon sugar substitute
1 clove garlic, crushed	1 teaspoon chili powder

Filling

¼ pound fresh spinach	2 cloves garlic, crushed
2 tablespoons olive oil	1 small fresh red chile, chopped
8 ears baby corn, sliced lengthwise	Salt and pepper
¼ cup peas, thawed if frozen	
½ cup diced red bell pepper	4 tortillas
½ cup peeled, diced carrot	12 ounces grated Cheddar cheese (about 1½ cups)
½ sliced leek (white part only), trimmed in quarter-inch rounds and thoroughly washed	

Combine all the sauce ingredients in a small, heavy saucepan. Bring to a boil, stirring constantly. Lower heat to medium and cook about 20 minutes until thick, stirring occasionally.

While the sauce is cooking, bring a pot of water to a boil. Add the spinach and cook 1 minute. Drain thoroughly and let cool, then chop coarsely. Preheat the oven to 350°.

Heat the oil in a skillet over medium heat. Add the corn, peas, bell pepper, carrot, leek, garlic, and chile. Cook for 3 to 4 minutes, stirring briskly. Do not let the vegetables brown. Stir in the spinach and season with salt and pepper.

Spoon one quarter of the filling in the center of each of the tortillas; roll up and place seam-side down in a single layer in a shallow baking dish. Pour the sauce over and sprinkle with the cheese. Bake about 25 minutes.

Serve with the salad of your choice.

TURKEY LASAGNA

SERVES 4

Cooking spray	1½ cups diced zucchini (½-inch pieces)
7 ounces ground turkey or turkey sausage, casing removed	⅓ cup low-fat or fat-free ricotta cheese
	1 tablespoon grated Parmesan cheese
1 medium onion, chopped	1 tablespoon chopped fresh parsley
1¾ cups spaghetti sauce	3 ounces grated reduced-fat mozzarella
⅔ cup water	cheese (about ¾ cup)
1½ cups wide egg noodles	

Lightly coat a large skillet with cooking spray. Brown the turkey over medium-high heat, stirring to break up lumps. Add the onion and cook until tender. Drain off excess fat. Add the spaghetti sauce and water. Bring to a boil and add the noodles. Cook for 3 minutes, then add the zucchini. Bring back to a boil, reduce heat and simmer about 10 minutes, stirring occasionally, until noodles are tender.

Mix the ricotta, Parmesan, and parsley in a small bowl; stir until a smooth paste forms. Drop by rounded teaspoonfuls onto the simmering mixture, making 10 to 12 small mounds. Sprinkle the mozzarella evenly over all, reduce the heat to low, and cook 4 to 5 minutes more. Let stand 10 minutes before serving.

Enjoy with a mixed green salad of your choice.

VEGETABLE LASAGNA

SERVES 4

Salt	½ cup low-fat cottage cheese
4 lasagna noodles	2 tablespoons grated Parmesan cheese
2 teaspoons olive oil	⅛ teaspoon ground black pepper
2 cups zucchini or yellow squash in ¼-inch crosswise slices	Cooking spray
	1¾ cups spaghetti sauce
1½ cups sliced mushrooms	⅔ cup shredded low-fat mozzarella cheese
⅓ cup chopped onions	1 medium tomato, sliced into ¼-inch rounds
⅔ cup light ricotta cheese	

Bring a large pot of salted water to a boil; cook the noodles according to package directions. Drain and rinse with cold water. Set aside. While the noodles are cooking, preheat the oven to 350°.

Heat the oil in a large skillet over medium heat; add the squash, mushrooms, and onion. Cook 4 to 5 minutes, until tender. Set aside.

Combine the ricotta, cottage cheese, Parmesan, and pepper in a small bowl.

Lightly coat a 9½ by 6-inch glass baking dish with cooking spray. Place 2 noodles in the bottom in a single layer. Evenly spread half the cheese mixture over the noodles; top with half the vegetables, half the sauce, and half of the mozzarella. Repeat with the remaining noodles, cheese mixture, vegetables, and sauce.

Bake uncovered about 30 minutes. Arrange the tomato slices on top and sprinkle with the remaining mozzarella. Return to the oven for 5 minutes more, until everything is thoroughly heated. Let stand 10 minutes before serving.

Serve with a mixed green salad.

SALMON STEAKS WITH LIME BUTTER AND ASPARAGUS RICE

SERVES 4

Lime butter

4 teaspoons butter, at room temperature	4 salmon steaks, 3 ounces each, with skin and bones removed
1 tablespoon chopped fresh cilantro	
1 teaspoon finely grated lime zest	1 teaspoon Sugar Ranch "MŌcean" fennel pollen spice blend
1½ teaspoons fresh lime juice	
Salt and pepper	

In a small bowl, thoroughly combine the butter, cilantro, lime zest and juice, and salt and pepper to make the lime butter. Roll into a silver dollar–diameter log using waxed paper, and refrigerate.

Preheat the broiler. Season the salmon steaks with the fennel pollen blend. Broil the salmon steaks for 5 minutes on each side, until opaque and flaky. While the salmon is cooking, make the Asparagus Rice (recipe follows).

Slice the lime butter into 4 portions. Place 1 portion on each salmon steak, and serve the asparagus rice alongside.

Asparagus Rice

Cooking spray	1 teaspoon finely grated fresh ginger
½ pound fresh asparagus, trimmed and cut diagonally into 1-inch pieces	½ cup drained sliced water chestnuts
	3 tablespoons soy sauce
1 cup sliced fresh shiitake mushroom caps	Pepper
2 cups cooked rice (from ⅔ cup raw regular rice or 1 cup instant)	

Lightly coat a skillet with cooking spray. Stir-fry the asparagus and mushrooms about 3 minutes, until well heated. Add the rice and ginger, and stir-fry for 2 minutes more. Add the water chestnuts and soy sauce and stir-fry for 1 minute longer. Season with pepper.

SCALLOP KABOBS

SERVES 4

1 (8-ounce) can pineapple chunks in natural juice	8 snow pea pods
½ pound large sea scallops (8 pieces)	8 cherry tomatoes
½ teaspoon ground ginger	1 zucchini, cut into eight 1-inch pieces
1 fresh red chile, seeded and chopped	4 skewers
Juice and grated zest of 1 lemon	

Drain the pineapple and set aside the chunks. In a medium glass or plastic bowl, combine the pineapple juice, scallops, ginger, chile, and lemon juice and zest. Cover and marinate at room temperature for 20 minutes or in the refrigerator for 2 hours.

Bring a pot of water to a boil. Add the snow peas and cook for 30 seconds, just until they are pliable. Drain and rinse under cold water.

Preheat the broiler or barbecue.

Drain the scallops and reserve the marinade. Wrap a snow pea around a scallop and thread it onto a skewer. Thread a cherry tomato, piece of zucchini, chunk of pineapple, then repeat with another snow pea–wrapped scallop, tomato, and pieces of zucchini and pineapple. Repeat with the remaining skewers.

Broil 3 inches from the heat (or barbecue), basting frequently with the marinade and turning occasionally. Cook for about 5 minutes.

Serve with rice and a tossed salad.

Notes: If you like, you can use 8 peeled, deveined extra-large shrimp, or swordfish cut into eight 1-inch cubes, instead.

Soak bamboo skewers in water for an hour beforehand so they won't burn.

Other veggies can be added or substituted, such as onion, bell pepper, or mushrooms. Additional veggie skewers can be made and cooked at the same.

CHEESE-STUFFED PASTA SHELLS

SERVES 4

Salt	¼ cup water
12 jumbo pasta shells	1 cup part-skim ricotta
Cooking spray	⅓ cup finely shredded Romano or Parmesan cheese (about 1¼ ounces)
1 tablespoon olive oil	
1 cup chopped onion	1 tablespoon finely chopped fresh basil
1 cup chopped fennel (1 small bulb)	1 (26-ounce) jar marinara sauce
2 cloves garlic, minced	¼ cup dry red wine (optional)
1½ cups chopped broccoli	1½ teaspoon fennel seeds, crushed

Bring a large pot of salted water to a boil and cook the pasta according to the package directions. Drain, rinse with cold water, and drain again. Set aside.

Preheat the oven to 375°. Lightly coat a 2-quart rectangular baking dish with cooking spray and set aside.

Heat the oil in a large nonstick skillet over medium-high heat. Add the onion, fennel, and garlic and cook, stirring occasionally for 3–6 minutes, until almost tender. Add the broccoli and water. Cover and cook over medium-low heat about 5 minutes, until the vegetables are tender. Remove from the heat. Drain. Stir the cheeses and basil into the vegetables.

Spoon the vegetable-cheese mixture into the cooked pasta shells. Spread ½ cup of the marinara sauce evenly in the bottom of the baking dish. Arrange the stuffed shells on top. Combine the remaining sauce, wine, and fennel seeds. Spoon over the shells. Cover loosely with foil and bake about 35 minutes, until cheese is melted and sauce is bubbly.

Serve with a green salad.

STUFFED GREEN PEPPERS

SERVES 4

4 medium green bell peppers	½ teaspoon dried basil or oregano
Cooking spray	¼ teaspoon salt
12 ounces lean ground beef or ground turkey	¼ teaspoon ground black pepper
½ cup chopped red onion	2 peeled, seeded, chopped tomatoes (a little more than 1 cup)
1½ cups water	¼ cup grated Cheddar or Jack cheese (about 1 ounce)
½ cup long-grain rice	
1 tablespoon Worcestershire sauce	

Bring a large pot of water to a boil; fill a large bowl with ice and water. Cut the tops off the peppers and remove the seeds. Immerse the peppers in the boiling water for 3 minutes. Remove and cool in the ice water. Place the peppers upside down on paper towels to drain.

Preheat the oven to 375°.

Lightly coat a large skillet with cooking spray. Brown the meat over medium-high heat, stirring to break up lumps. Add the onion and cook until tender. Drain off excess fat. Add the water, rice, Worcestershire sauce, basil, salt, and pepper. Bring to a boil, reduce heat, cover and simmer about 15 minutes, stirring occasionally, until the rice is tender. Stir in the tomatoes.

Lightly coat an 8 by 8-inch baking dish with cooking spray. Place the peppers upright so they don't tip over. Spoon the meat mixture into the peppers. Bake for 20 minutes. Remove from the oven and sprinkle with the cheese. Let stand until the cheese is melted.

Serve with a mixed green salad.

TURKEY CHILI

SERVES 5

Cooking spray	4 stalks celery, diced
12 ounces ground turkey	1 package chili seasoning mix
2 green bell peppers, diced	4 (14.5-ounce) cans stewed tomatoes
1 medium onion, chopped	1 (15-ounce) can black beans, drained
2 medium zucchini or yellow squash, chopped	2 cups low-fat beef or chicken broth
	Salt and pepper

Lightly coat a medium skillet with cooking spray. Brown the turkey over medium-high heat, stirring to break up lumps. Drain off fat and set aside.

Lightly coat a large soup pot with cooking spray, and sauté the bell peppers, onions, squash, and celery. When the vegetables are almost tender but still a little crunchy, add the chili mix, tomatoes, beans, broth, turkey, and salt and pepper. Simmer for 30 minutes, stirring occasionally.

Notes: If you want it a little spicier, add more chili mix.

This recipe gets the best results cooked in a large quantity. It freezes well, so freeze individual portions for your next chili craving!!!

Add one cup of cooked vegetables or small salad with non-fat dressing.

OVEN-FRIED FISH WITH COLESLAW

SERVES 4

Cooking spray	2 tablespoons grated Parmesan cheese
1 pound skinless fish fillets (any kind)	¼ teaspoon lemon-pepper seasoning
¼ cup nonfat milk	1 tablespoon melted butter
⅓ cup all-purpose flour	
½ cup crushed Uncle Sam Cereal® or dry bread crumbs	

Preheat the oven to 450°. Lightly coat a shallow baking dish with cooking spray.

Cut the fish into 4 serving-size portions. Place the milk in one shallow dish and the flour in a second. In a third, mix the cereal, cheese, lemon pepper, and butter.

Dip each piece of fish first in the milk, then the flour; shake off any excess. Dip the fish in milk again and finally in the cereal mixture. Press the crumbs on to coat all sides.

Lay the fish in the baking dish in one layer. Bake uncovered until the fish flakes, about 5 minutes for every ¼-inch of thickness.

Serve the fish with the Coleslaw (recipe follows).

Coleslaw

SERVES 8, 1 CUP PER SERVING

1 small head cabbage, shredded	2 tablespoons white vinegar
2 cups shredded carrots	3 tablespoons apple juice
2 stalks celery, shredded	½ cup nonfat unflavored yogurt
¼ cup raisins	Salt and pepper
1 cup peeled, cored, diced apple (1 large apple)	

In a medium bowl, combine the cabbage, carrots, celery, raisins, and apple. In a small bowl, whisk together the vinegar, juice, and yogurt. Pour the dressing over the vegetables, season with salt and pepper, and mix well. (If making the coleslaw ahead, cover and refrigerate it until serving time.)

ROSEMARY LAMB CHOPS

SERVES 4

2 tablespoons olive oil	½ cup low-sugar apricot or peach jam
2 teaspoons chopped fresh rosemary or ½ teaspoon dried rosemary	¼ cup water
	1 tablespoon Dijon mustard
½ teaspoon ground black pepper	1 chicken bouillon cube
2 cloves garlic, minced	½ teaspoon chopped fresh mint
8 lamb rib chops (1 to ½ pounds), fat trimmed	

Combine 1 tablespoon of the oil, the rosemary, pepper, and garlic in a small bowl. Brush this mixture onto all sides of the chops. Set aside.

In a small saucepan, prepare a glaze by combining the jam, water, mustard, bouillon cube, and mint. Bring to a boil, stirring. Remove from the heat, and set aside to keep warm.

Heat the remaining tablespoon of oil in a large skillet over medium heat. Add the chops. Cook about 3 minutes on each side, until desired doneness (medium is 160° on an instant-read thermometer).

Serve with the glaze, ½ cup of rice pilaf per serving, and a mixed green salad of choice.

CHICKEN BAKE WITH RAW BROCCOLI SALAD

SERVES 4

Cooking spray	½ teaspoon fennel seeds, crushed
⅓ cup nonfat dry milk powder	1 tablespoon low-sodium chicken-flavor bouillon granules
1 teaspoon salt	
½ teaspoon ground black pepper	4 skinless, boneless chicken breasts (4 ounces each)
½ teaspoon dry mustard	
2 teaspoons paprika	Water

Preheat the oven to 400°. Lightly coat a shallow baking dish with cooking spray.

Mix the milk, salt, pepper, mustard, paprika, fennel seeds, and bouillon granules in a plastic bag. Dip the chicken in water, then shake individually in the bag of coating. Lay the chicken in the baking dish in one layer. Bake for 25 minutes.

Serve with Raw Broccoli Salad (recipe follows) and a dinner roll.

Raw Broccoli Salad

4 cups broccoli florets, chopped into small pieces	1 tablespoon Splenda® or 1 teaspoon other sugar substitute
¼ cup minced red onion	2 teaspoons cider vinegar
3 tablespoons golden raisins	2 teaspoons raw sunflower seeds
2 tablespoons light mayonnaise	

Place the broccoli, onion, and raisins in a medium bowl. In a small bowl, whisk the mayonnaise, sugar substitute, and vinegar until combined. Pour over the broccoli and toss to mix well. Sprinkle with the sunflower seeds. Chill before serving.

TOFU STIR-FRY

SERVES 4

1 cup quick-cooking brown rice	½ teaspoon red pepper flakes (optional)
½ cup vegetable or chicken broth	Cooking spray
¼ cup dry sherry	1 cup thinly sliced carrots, cut on the bias
1 tablespoon cornstarch	2 cloves garlic, minced
1 tablespoon reduced-sodium soy sauce	2 cups broccoli florets
1 teaspoon sugar substitute	2 cups ½-inch cubes of firm tofu
1 teaspoon grated fresh ginger	

Prepare the rice according to package directions and keep warm.

In a small bowl, stir together the broth, sherry, cornstarch, sugar substitute, ginger, and pepper flakes. Set aside.

Lightly coat a wok or large skillet with cooking spray. Heat over medium-high heat. Add the carrots and garlic and stir-fry for 2 minutes without browning. Add the broccoli and stir-fry for 3 to 4 minutes more, until the vegetables are crisp-tender. Push the vegetables to the side of the wok. Add the sauce to the middle of the wok and stir until thickened and bubbly. Add the tofu and stir all ingredients to coat. Cook for 1 minute more.

To serve, spoon each portion over ½ cup of cooked brown rice.

EASY CHICKEN AND VEGETABLES

SERVES 4

4 small red or white new potatoes	1 (10-ounce) package frozen cut green beans, thawed
1½ tablespoons butter	
½ cup chopped shallots	½ teaspoon Sugar Ranch "Salt-Free Heaven" fennel pollen spice blend
1 teaspoon chopped garlic	
12 ounces skinless, boneless chicken breasts, cut into small strips	Salt and pepper

Boil or microwave the potatoes until just tender; set aside and keep warm.

Meanwhile, melt the butter in a heavy skillet over medium heat. Add the shallots and garlic. Stir and cook for 3 minutes. Remove and set aside. Place the chicken in the skillet and cook about 10 minutes, until cooked through. Remove the chicken from the skillet and keep warm. Return the shallots to the skillet with the green beans and pepper, and turn the heat down to medium-low. Cover and cook about 5 minutes, until the beans are tender. Add the chicken and potatoes and cook 3 to 4 minutes, stirring occasionally, until heated. Sprinkle with the fennel pollen spices and season with salt and pepper.

SLOW COOKER TURKEY BREAST

SERVES 4

1 whole turkey breast	1 cup boiling water
2 small boxes sugar-free cranberry gelatin	1 small packet dry onion soup mix

Place the turkey breast skin-side up in the slow cooker. Dissolve the gelatin in the boiling water and pour over the turkey. Sprinkle the onion soup mix over all. Cover and cook on HIGH for 3 hours. Reduce heat to LOW and cook for 3 hours more, until the turkey is tender.

BAKED CHICKEN AND CHIPS

SERVES 4

4 small baking potatoes, scrubbed and dried	8 chicken drumsticks, skin removed
1 tablespoon olive oil	1 whole egg
1 teaspoon sea salt or kosher salt	2 tablespoons water
1 tablespoon all-purpose flour	6 tablespoons crushed Uncle Sam Cereal® or dry bread crumbs
Pinch of cayenne pepper	
½ teaspoon paprika	Salt and pepper
½ teaspoon dried thyme	

Preheat the oven to 400°.

Follow these helpful suggestions to lighten up your traditional holiday meals. Holiday meals don't have to be packed with calories to taste good.

- Baked turkey—choose a plain bird over a self-basting bird to lower the sodium content. To ensure a moist bird, bake unstuffed, leave the skin on while roasting and remove from the oven when internal temperature reaches 170° in the breast (check with an instant-read thermometer).
- Gravy—use a gravy cup or refrigerate the pan juices (to harden the fat) and skim the fat off before making gravy. This saves around 56 grams of fat per cup.
- Dressing—use a little less bread and add more onions, celery, vegetables, or even fruits such as cranberries and apples.
- Candied yams—leave out the margarine and marshmallows. Sweeten with fruit juice such as apple, and flavor with cinnamon.
- Green bean casserole—cook fresh green beans with chunks of potatoes instead of cream soup. Top with sliced or slivered almonds instead of fried onion rings.
- Mashed potatoes—use skim milk, garlic powder, and a little Parmesan cheese instead of whole milk and butter.
- Pumpkin pie
- Rolls—serve smaller rolls or leave them out completely.

Cut each potato lengthwise into 8 equal wedges. Place in a plastic bag, add the oil, and shake well to coat. Arrange skin-side down on a nonstick baking sheet, sprinkle with the sea salt, and bake for 30 to 35 minutes until tender and golden.

Meanwhile, mix the flour, cayenne, paprika, thyme, and salt and pepper together in a shallow bowl. Lightly beat the egg and water in a second shallow bowl. In a third, sprinkle the cereal.

Dip each piece of chicken first in the flour; shake off any excess. Dip the chicken next in the eggs, and finally in the cereal. Press the crumbs on to coat all sides.

Place the chicken on the baking sheet with the potato wedges and bake for 30 minutes, turning after 15 minutes. Remove when the potatoes and chicken are tender and cooked thoroughly.

Serve with steamed vegetables and tossed salad.

TURKEY MEATBALL PITAS

SERVES 4

½ (12-ounce) package fully cooked turkey meatballs

1 teaspoon ground cumin

1 teaspoon paprika

1 cup peeled, diced cucumber

1 cup unflavored yogurt

1 tablespoon fresh lemon juice

2 tablespoons finely chopped fresh dill

¼ teaspoon salt

4 small pitas

4 large lettuce leaves of choice (such as romaine or red-leaf)

8 thin slices tomato, halved

Fresh dill

Heat the meatballs in a microwave-safe dish as directed on the package. Halfway through, sprinkle with ½ teaspoon of the cumin and ½ teaspoon of the paprika. Stir often.

While the meatballs are heating, mix the cucumber, yogurt, lemon juice, dill, salt, and the remaining cumin and paprika in a small bowl.

On top of each pita, arrange 1 lettuce leaf and 4 pieces of tomato. Top with the meatballs (cut in half if you wish). Spoon the cucumber sauce over all.

Lunch/Dinner: Frozen Meals

Many frozen meals do not come with a large vegetable serving, so we have created the salads below for your enjoyment and to complete a balanced, nutritional meal.

For all Lunch & Dinner options choose from the following salads:

If cheese is not in your frozen meal, choose from the following selections of salads:

- Add a large romaine lettuce salad complete with ½ cup of boiled artichoke hearts, ½ cup steamed green beans, and 1 ounce of Monterey Jack cheese. Drizzle with 1 tablespoon of low-fat or nonfat dressing, or use 1 teaspoon of flax oil with a squeeze of lemon.
- Add a large spinach salad with 1 ounce of feta cheese and 1 cup steamed and sliced eggplant. Drizzle with 1 tablespoon of low-fat

or nonfat balsamic dressing, or 1 teaspoon of flax oil with a squeeze of lemon.

If your frozen meal does include cheese, choose from the following selections of salads:

- Add a large iceberg lettuce salad with 1 medium tomato (sliced or cubed) and 1 cup of an assortment of sliced bell peppers. Drizzle with 1 tablespoon of low-fat or nonfat dressing or use 1 teaspoon of flax oil with a squeeze of lemon.
- Add a large spinach salad with whole or sliced mushrooms and a sprinkle of radish slices. Drizzle with 1 tablespoon of low-fat or nonfat balsamic dressing or 1 teaspoon of flax oil with a squeeze of lemon.

Lean Cuisine® Café Classics Chicken Carbonara

Lean Cuisine® Cheese Cannelloni

Lean Cuisine® Café Classics Cheese Lasagna with Chicken Scaloppini

Lean Cuisine® Dinnertime Selections Salisbury Steak

Healthy Choice® Rigatoni w/ Broccoli and Chicken

Healthy Choice® Flavor Adventures Roasted Chicken Chardonnay

Healthy Choice® Oven Roasted Beef

Healthy Choice® Roasted Chicken Breast

Weight Watchers®, Smart Ones®, Ham & Cheddar Smartwich

Weight Watchers®, Smart Ones®, Deluxe Pizza

Weight Watchers®, Smart Ones®, Lemon Herb Chicken Piccata

Weight Watchers®, Smart Ones®, Peppercorn Fillet of Beef

Amy's Kitchen® Spinach Feta in a Pocket Sandwich (1)

Amy's Kitchen® Stuffed Pasta Shells Bowl

Amy's Kitchen® Cheese Enchilada

Amy's Kitchen® Vegetable Lasagna

Lunch/Dinner: Fast Food

BAJA FRESH®

- Any choice of one (1) Baja Style Taco (Chicken, Steak or Gulf Shrimp). Add side salad with no dressing or squeeze of lime for flavor.
- 1 Fish Taco with Charbroiled Fish. Add side salad with a squeeze of lime or lemon.

BOSTON MARKET®

- Dark meat chicken quarter, without skin. Add a bowl of vegetable soup or a side of rice pilaf.
- Order of Honey Glazed Ham. Add 2 sides, New Potatoes and Green Beans, or Green Bean Casserole.

BURGER KING®

- Hamburger. Add side salad with fat-free or low-fat dressing or squeeze of lemon.
- Fire-Grilled Chicken or Shrimp Salad. Add fat-free or low-fat dressing and a packet of crackers if available.
- Whopper Jr. without mayonnaise. Add side Garden Salad w/Kraft® Fat-Free Ranch Dressing.

DAIRY QUEEN®

- BBQ Beef or Pork Sandwich. Add a side salad with nonfat or fat-free dressing.
- Grilled Chicken Salad with nonfat or fat-free dressing. Add package of crackers or a small roll.

DEL TACO®

- Two Chicken Tacos Del Carbon

EL POLLO LOCO®

- 1 leg and 1 thigh of Flame-Grilled Chicken. 1 (6-inch) corn tortilla and a corn cobette or fresh vegetables.

FAZOLI'S®

- Chicken & Pasta Caesar Salad. Add reduced calorie Italian dressing.

IN 'N' OUT BURGER®

- [Hamburger with onion protein style.] Ask for half order of french fries. Add mustard and ketchup instead of spread on burger.
- Hamburger with onion. Use mustard and ketchup instead of spread.

JACK IN THE BOX®

- Chicken Fajita Pita. Add 1 side salad, use lemon as dressing.
- Asian Chicken Salad. Use low-fat balsamic vinaigrette dressing and add 1 egg roll.

KFC®

- Chicken Breast without skin or breading. Add order of green beans or 3-inch corn on the cob with order of mashed potatoes without gravy; add pat of butter.

MCDONALD'S®

- 1 Cheeseburger. Add side salad with low-fat balsamic vinaigrette
- 1 Bacon Ranch Salad without chicken. Add a Fruit N' Yogurt Parfait with or without granola for dessert.
- Egg McMuffin. Add 1 glass of 1% milk.
- Chicken McGrill. Add a side salad, use lemon as dressing or Newman's Own Low Fat Balsamic Vinaigrette (use only half the packet).

SONIC®

- Grilled Chicken Sandwich.
- Grilled Chicken Wrap without ranch dressing.

SUBWAY®

- 6-inch Ham without mayo. Salt, pepper, and mustard optional. Add salad with choice of lemon squeeze or Kraft fat-free Italian dressing or order of soup. Choose from the following: Roasted Chicken Noodle, Minestrone.

- 6" Turkey Breast without mayonnaise. Salt, pepper, and mustard optional. Add Garden Fresh Salad with choice of lemon squeeze or Kraft® Fat-Free Italian dressing, or order of soup. Choose from the following: Roasted Chicken Noodle or Minestrone.
- 6" Tuna Sandwich, open-faced. Add Garden Fresh Salad w/squeeze of lemon or Kraft® Fat-Free Italian dressing.

TACO BELL®

- All items ordered "fresco style"
- 2 Ranchero Chicken Soft Tacos.
- Beef, Chicken, or Steak Enchirito.
- Gordita Baja: Beef, Chicken, or Steak.
- 2 Grilled Steak Soft Tacos.

WENDY'S®

- 1 Jr. Hamburger. Add a side salad w. fat-free French dressing.
- Mandarin Chicken Salad. Add low-fat honey mustard dressing.
- Grilled Chicken Sandwich. Add caesar side salad with lemon squirt in place of dressing provided.
- Taco Supremo Salad. Use salsa as dressing.

NOTE: Visit JorgeCruise.com for the newest homemade, frozen, and fast-food ideas in our Success News section.

SNACKS

For each specified amount, fill in the snack line on your Cruise Timeline™. In general, your snacks are about 100 calories.

Almonds (12)

Angel food cake (2-ounce slice)

Baby carrots (2 cups)

Baker's® cookie (www. bbcookies.com) (1)

Breadsticks, 4 inch long (2)

Brownie, small (1)

Butterscotch (4 pieces)

Candy corn (20 pieces)

Cashews (12)

Celery (3 stalks with 1 teaspoon of peanut butter on each)

Cheez-It® Twisterz (12)

Chips, baked, tortilla or potato (¾ ounce or 15 to 20 chips)

Chocolate-covered almonds (7)

Dannon® DanActive— Orange (1)

Dannon® DanActive— Original (1)

Dannon® DanActive— Strawberry (1)

Dannon® DanActive— Vanilla (1)

Dannon® Light'n Fit Creamy, all flavors (6 oz.)

Dannon® Light'n Fit Smoothie, all flavors (1 bottle)

Dannon® Light'n Fit Yogurt, all flavors (6 oz.)

Earthbound Farm Organic Snack Pack: Carrots with Ranch Dip

Fruit, 1 piece (see fruit lists in chapter 12 for portion size)

Fudge (1 ounce)

Gelatin (½ cup)

GeniSoy® Soy Crisps (25)

Goldfish® Crisps, Four Cheese (25)

Graham crackers, 2½-inch squares (3)

Granola bar, low-fat (1)

Gumdrops (1 ounce)

Handi-Snacks®, Mister Salty Pretzels n' Cheese (1 pack)

Heath® bar (1 snack size)

Hershey's® milk chocolate bar (1 small)

Hershey's® milk chocolate bar with almonds (1 small)

Hershey's® Sweet Escapes (1 bar, any kind)

Jell-O® Smoothie Snacks, all flavors (1 snack)

Kellogg's® Cocoa Rice Krispies Bar (1)

Kellogg's® Tony's Cinnamon Krunchers Bar (1)

Kit Kat® (one 2-piece bar)

Knudsen® On the Go!
Low-fat Cottage Cheese
(1 serving)

Kudos® with M&M's granola
bar (1)

Melba toast (4 slices)

Mott's® Single Serve
Cinnamon Apple Sauce
(1 cup)

Mott's® Single Serve
Strawberry Apple Sauce
(1 cup)

Nabisco® 100 Calorie Pack,
Chips Ahoy! Thin crisps
(1 bag)

Nabisco® 100 Calorie Pack,
Fruit Snacks Mixed Berry
(1 bag)

Nabisco® 100 Calorie Pack,
Kraft Cheese Nips thin
crisps (1 bag)

Nabisco® 100 Calorie Pack,
Oreo thin crisps (1 bag)

Nabisco® 100 Calorie Pack,
Wheat Thins minis (1 bag)

Nabisco® Ritz Chips,
Cheddar (10 chips)

Nabisco® Ritz Chips, Regular
(10 chips)

Nabisco® Ritz Chips, Sour
Cream & Onion (10 chips)

Nature Valley® Granola Bar,
all flavors (1 bar)

No Pudge! Fat Free Fudge
Brownie (www.nopudge.
com) (one 2-inch square)

Orville Redenbacher's®
Popcorn Mini Cakes, all
flavors (10 cakes)

Oyster crackers (24)

Peanut brittle (1 ounce)

Peanuts (20)

Pecans (8 halves)

Popcorn, air popped (3 cups)

Potato chips, fat-free (15–20)

Pound cake (1-ounce slice)

Pretzels (¾ ounce)

Pria® Bar, all flavors, (1 bar)

Pringles® Reduced Fat
Original, 8 pack (1 pack)

Pudding cup, fat-free (1)

Pumpkin seeds (2
tablespoons)

Quaker® Quakes Corn Rings,
BBQ (20)

Quaker® Quakes Corn Rings,
Cheddar Cheese (20)

Quaker® Quakes Corn Rings,
Nacho Cheese (20)

Raisins (30)

Rice cakes (2)

Saltine crackers (6)

Sargento®, Cheeze & Sticks
Snacks (1 pack)

Sesame seeds (2
tablespoons)

Sherbet (½ cup)

Skinny Cow® fat-free fudge
bar (1)

Skinny Cow® low-fat ice
cream sandwich (½)

Soda crackers (4)

Stretch Island Fruit Leather,
Any Flavor (2)

String cheese (1)

Sunflower seeds (2
tablespoons)

Tofutti (¼ cup)

Tortilla chips, fat-free (15
to 20)

Trader Joe's Low-fat Rice
Crisps, Caramel (14 crisps)

Trader Joe's Low-fat White Cheddar Corn Crisps (20 crisps)

Uncle Sam Cereal® (½ cup dry)

Whole wheat crackers (2–5)

Whoppers malted milk balls (9)

Yogurt, frozen, low-fat or nonfat (½ cup)

TREATS

For each specified amount, fill in the treat line on your Cruise Timeline™.
Eat a delicious treat every day. In general, they should be 30 to 50 calories.

Animal crackers (4)
Caramel piece (2½-ounce piece)
Cheese slice, reduced-calorie (1)
Chocolate chips (½ tablespoon)
Chocolate-coated mints (4)
Cookie, butter (1)
Cookie, fat-free (1 small)
Cookie, fortune (1)
Corn cake (1)
Crackers, Triscuits® (2)
Cranberry sauce (¼ cup)
European chestnuts (1 ounce)
Frozen seedless grapes (1 cup)
Gelatin dessert, sugar-free (1)
Gingersnaps (3)
Ginkgo nuts (1 ounce or 14 medium)
Graham crackers (2½" square)
Gumdrops (2)
Hard candy (1)
Hershey's® Hugs or Kisses (2)
Hershey's® Miniatures (1, any kind)
Ice milk, vanilla (¼ cup)
Ice pop, made with water (2 ounce pop)
Jelly beans (7)

Licorice twist (1)
Life Savers, all fruit flavors (3)
Lollipop, Life [Savers,] swirled flavor (1)
M&M's® (¼ of small bag)
M&M's® Minis (¼ of tube)
Marshmallow (1 large)
Marshmallows, mini (¼ cup)
Miss Meringue cookie (www.missmeringue.com) (1)
Nonfat ice cream (½ cup) drizzled with Hershey's chocolate syrup
Oreo cookie (1)
Popcorn, air popped (1 cup)
Pretzels (½ ounce)
Prune (1)
Raisins (1 tablespoon)
Raisins, chocolate covered (10)
Reese's® Peanut Butter Cup (1)
Rice Krispies Treat square (½)
Ritz Bits® peanut butter (5)
SnackWell's® sandwich cookie (1)
Starburst®, fruit chew (1)
Stretch Island Fruit Leather, Any Flavor (1)
Teddy Grahams®, honey flavor (6)
Vanilla wafers (2)
York peppermint pattie (1 small)

JORGE CRUISE'S BIO

"America's newest weight-loss guru!"

—BETTER NUTRITION MAGAZINE

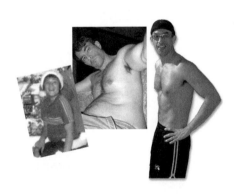

Jorge Cruise personally struggled with weight as a child and young man. Today he is recognized as America's leading weight-loss expert for busy people. He is the #1 *New York Times* best-selling author of *8 Minutes in the Morning*®, published in 14 languages. Jorge has also coached more than 3 million online clients at JorgeCruise.com and is the exclusive weight-loss coach for AOL's 23 million subscribers. Each Sunday his "USA Weekend" column is read by more than 50 million readers in 600 newspapers nationwide. Jorge is also *First for Women* magazine's "Slimming Coach" columnist with more than 3 million readers each month. He has appeared on *Oprah*, CNN, *Good Morning America*, the *Today* show, *Dateline NBC*, and *The View*.

Utilizing the knowledge and credentials that he has gained from the University of California, San Diego (UCSD), Dartmouth College, the Cooper Institute for Aerobics Research, the American College of Sports Medicine

(ACSM), and the American Council on Exercise (ACE), Jorge is dedicated to helping busy people lose weight without fad dieting.

Jorge lives in San Diego, California, with his wife, Heather, and son, Parker. He can be contacted via JorgeCruise.com or AOL keyword Jorge Cruise.

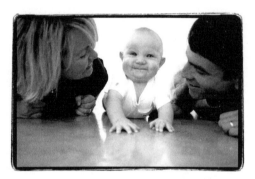

THE CRUISE FAMILY: HEATHER, BABY PARKER, AND JORGE

"Jorge Cruise has answers that really work and take almost no time. I recommend them highly."

—ANDREW WEIL, MD,

DIRECTOR OF THE PROGRAM IN

INTEGRATIVE MEDICINE, UNIVERSITY OF ARIZONA

The 3-Hour Diet™
Additional Tools

Want to get the most out of *The 3-Hour Diet*™? Check out these ways to take your plan to the next level.

JorgeCruise.com

Sometimes staying motivated and organized can get complicated. Guarantee your success by staying connected to Jorge Cruise and his LIVE mentors to ensure you lose two pounds every week with the 3-Hour Diet™. Having this kind of support can be the difference between reaching the finish line and running in place.

Join our club and you'll get:

1. A personalized weekly 3-hour meal planner that will make eating on time automatic and effortless.

2. Delicious recipes you can make at home in minutes from real foods—including carbs! New recipes added each month.

3. Frozen food options from brand names like: Lean Cuisine®, Healthy Choice®, Amy's Kitchen®

4. Fast-food options from:

McDonald's®	KFC®
Arby's®	Subway®
In 'N' Out®	Taco Bell®
Burger King®	(and many more)
Jack in the Box®	

Plus you get access to our support boards, online meetings, buddy system, and daily audio coaching direct from Jorge to keep you motivated. Joining our club is like joining a family. Imagine no deprivation, the end to low-carb dieting, and two pounds gone every week by eating!

Visit JorgeCruise.com and get a FREE 3-Hour Diet™ profile today.

More Support Tools

The 3-Hour Diet™ **Audio**

Experience the 3-Hour Diet™ revolution direct from Jorge Cruise. On his exclusive audio program he will walk you through all the secrets of how to lose two pounds a week without any deprivation or fad dieting. As an added bonus you will also hear actual success interviews with the 3-Hour Diet™ clients. Get ready to boost your motivation and success to the highest levels! Available everywhere books are sold.

The 3-Hour Diet™ **Book in Spanish**

Jorge's edition in Spanish has an inspirational foreword written by TV talk show host Cristina from *El Show de Cristina*. This version is perfect for the Spanish-speaking loved one in your life. Available everywhere books are sold.

The 3-Hour Diet™ **Journal**
The 3-Hour Diet™ **Cookbook**
The 3-Hour Diet™ **Eating Out Guide**

All coming out in 2006. For release dates and information, visit JorgeCruise .com.

8 Minutes in the Morning® **Book Series**

Want to accelerate your results? Then make sure to get Jorge's exercise book series. These toning and firming books are used at home to restore lost muscle, thus revving your metabolism even higher. And they only take eight minutes a day! Available everywhere books are sold.

SELECTED BIBLIOGRAPHY

Antoine, J. M., R. Rohr, M. J. Gagery, R. E. Bleyer, and G. Debry. "Feeding Frequency and Nitrogen Balance in Weight-reduction Obese Women." *Human Nutrition: Clinical Nutrition* 38 no. 1 (1984): 313–38.

"A Randomized Controlled Trial of 4 Different Commercial Weight Loss Programs in the UK in Obese Adults: Body Composition Changes over 6 Months." *Asia Pacific Journal of Clinical Nutrition.* 13: S146.

Astrup, A., T. Meinert Larsen, A. Harper. "Atkins and Other Low-carbohydrate Diets: Hoax or an Effective Tool for Weight Loss?" *Lancet.* 364 no. 9437: 897–99, 2004.

Bravata, D. M., L. Sanders, J. Huang, H. M. Krumholz, I. Olkin, C. D. Gardner, D. M. Bravata. "Efficacy and Safety of Low-carbohydrate Diets: A Systematic Review." *Journal of the American Medical Association.* 289 no. 14: 1837–50, 2003.

Butki, B. "Effects of a Carbohydrate-restricted Diet on Affective Responses to Acute Exercise among Physically Active Participants." *Perceptual and Motor Skills.* 96 no. 2 (2003): 607–15.

Crovetti, R., M. Porrini, A. Santangelo, and G. Testolin. "The Influence of the Thermic Effect of Food on Satiety." *European Journal of Clinical Nutrition.* 52 no. 7 (1998): 482–88.

de Jonge, L., and G. A. Bray. "The Thermic Effect of Food and Obesity: A Critical Review." *Obesity Research.* 5 no. 6 (1997): 622–31.

Deutz, R. C., D. Benardot, D. E. Martin, and M. M. Cody. "Relationship Between Energy Deficits and Body Composition in Elite Female Gymnasts and Runners." *Medicine and Science in Sports and Exercise.* 32 no.2 (2000): 659–68.

"Eat More Often to Combat Overeating." *Environmental Nutrition.* 23 no. 4 (2000): 8.

Farshchi, H. R., M. A. Taylor, and I. A. Macdonald. "Decreased Thermic Effect of Food after an Irregular Compared with a Regular Meal Pattern in Healthy Lean Women." *International Journal of Obesity Related Metabolic Disorders.* 28 no. 5 (2004): 653–60.

Farshchi, H. R., M. A. Taylor, and I. A. Macdonald. "Regular Meal Frequency Creates More Appropriate Insulin Sensitivity and Lipid Profiles Compared with Irregular Meal Frequency in Healthy Lean Women." *European Journal of Clinical Nutrition*. 58 no. 7 (2004): 1071–77.

Fogteloo, A. J., H. Pijl, F. Roelfsema, M. Frölich, and A. E. Meinders. "Impact of Meal Timing and Frequency on the Twenty-four-hour Leptin Rhythm." *Hormone Research*. 62 no. 2 (2004): 71–78.

Foster, G. D., H. R. Wyatt, J. O. Hill, B. G. McGuckin, C. Brill, B. S. Mohammed, P. O. Szapary, D. J. Rader, J. S. Edman, S. Klein. "A Randomized Trial of a Low-carbohydrate Diet for Obesity." *New England Journal of Medicine*. 22 no. 21 (2003): 2082–90.

Garrow, J. S., M. Durrant, S. Blaza, D. Wilkins, P. Royston, and S. Sunkin. "The Effect of Meal Frequency and Protein Concentration on the Composition of the Weight Lost by Obese Subjects." *British Journal of Nutrition*. 45 no.1 (1981): 5–15.

Gwinup, G., R. C. Byron, W. H. Roush, P. A. Kruger, and G. J. Hamwi. "Effect of Nibbling vs. Gorging on Cardiovascular Risk Factors: Serum Uric Acid and Blood Lipids." *Metabolism*. 44 no. 4 (1995): 549–55.

Hargreaves M. "Muscle Glycogen and Metabolic Regulation." *Proceedings of the Nutrition Society*. 63 no. 2: 217–20, 2004.

Hargreaves, M., J. Hawley, and A. Jeukendrup. "Pre Exercise Carbohydrate and Fat Ingestion: Effects on Metabolism and Performance." *Journal of Sports Sciences*. 22 no. 1: 31–38, 2004.

Hays, N. P., R. D. Starling, X. Liu, D. H. Sullivan, T. A. Trappe, J. D. Fluckey, and W. J. Evans. "Effects of an Ad Libitum Low-Fat, High-Carbohydrate Diet on Body Weight, Body Composition, and Fat Distribution in Older Men and Women: A Randomized Controlled Trial." *Archives of Internal Medicine*. 164 no. 2 (2004): 210–17.

Iwao, S., K. Mori, and Y. Sato. "Effects of Meal Frequency on Body Composition During Weight Control in Boxers." *Scandinavia Journal of Medicine & Science in Sports*. 6 no. 5 (1996): 265–72.

Jenkins, D. J., A. Ocana, A. L. Jenkins, T. M. Wolever, V. Vuksan, L. Katzman, M. Hollands, G. Greenberg, P. Corey, and R. Patten. "Metabolic Advantages of Spreading the Nutrient Load: Effects of Increased Meal Frequency in Non-insulin-dependent Diabetes." *American Journal of Clinical Nutrition*. 55 no. 2 (1992): 461–67.

Jenkins, D. J., T. M. Wolever, V. Vuksan, F. Brighen, S. C. Cunnane, A. V. Rao, et al. "Nibbling vs. Gorging: Metabolic Advantages of Increased Meal Frequency." *New England Journal of Medicine*. 321 no. 14 (1989): 929–34.

Kappagoda, C. T., D. A. Hyson, and E. A. Amsterdam. "Low-carbohydrate High-protein Diets: Is There a Place for Them in Clinical Cardiology?" *Journal of the American College of Cardiology*. 3 no. 43: 725–30, 2004.

Klem, M. L., R. R. Wing, M. T. McGuire, H. M. Seagle, and J. Hill. "A Descriptive Study of Individuals Successful at Long-term Maintenance of Substantial Weight Loss." *American Journal of Clinical Nutrition*. 66 no.2 (1997): 239–46.

Kwiterovich Jr., P. O., E. P. G. Vining, P. Pyzik, R. Skolasky Jr., and J. M. Freeman. "Effect of a High Fat Ketogenic Diet on Plasma Levels of Lipids, Lipoproteins, and

Apolipoproteins in Children." *Journal of the American Medical Association.* 290 no. 7: 912–20, 2003.

Landers, P., M. M. Wolfe, S. Glore, R. Guild, and L. Phillips. "Effect of Weight Loss Plans on Body Composition and Diet Duration." *Journal of the Oklahoma State Medical Association.* 95 no. 5: 329–31, 2002.

LeBlanc, J., I. Mercier, and A. Nadeau. "Components of Postprandial Thermognesis in Relation to Meal Frequency in Humans." *Canadian Journal of Physiology and Pharmacology.* 71 no. 12 (1993): 879–83.

Romon, M., P. Lebel, C. Velly, N. Marecaux, J. C. Fruchart, and J. Dallongeville. "Leptin Response to Carbohydrate or Fat Meal and Association with Subsequent Satiety and Energy Intake." *American Journal of Physiology.* 277 no. 5 (1999): E855–61.

Speechly, D. P., and R. Buffenstein. "Acute Appetite Reduction Associated with an Increased Frequency of Eating in Obese Males." *International Journal of Obesity Related Metabolic Disorders.* 23 no. 11 (1999): 1151–59.

Speechly, D. P., and R. Buffenstein. "Greater Appetite Control Associated with an Increased Frequency of Eating in Lean Males." *New England Journal of Medicine.* 321 no. 14 (1989): 929–34.

Venkatraman, J. T., and D. R. Pendergast. "Effect of Dietary Intake on Immune Function in Athletes." *Sports Medicine.* 32 no. 5: 323–37, 2002.

Verboeket-van de Venne, W. P., and K. R. Westerterp. "Influence of the Feeding Frequency on Nutrient Utilization in Man: Consequences for Energy Metabolism." *European Journal of Clinical Nutrition.* 45 no. 3 (1991): 161–69.

Wurtman, R. J., J. J. Wurtman, M. M. Regan, J. M. McDermott, R. H. Tsay, and J. J. Breu. "Effects of Normal Meals Rich in Carbohydrates or Proteins on Plasma Tryptophan and Tyrosine Ratios." *American Journal of Clinical Nutrition.* 77 no. 1 (2003): 128–32.

Yancy Jr., W. S., M. K. Olsen, J. R. Guyton, R. P. Bakst, and E. C. Westman. "A Low-carbohydrate Ketogenic Diet Versus a Low-fat Diet to Treat Obesity and Hyperlipidemia: A Randomized, Controlled Trial." *Annals of Internal Medicine.* 140 no. 10: 769–77, 2004.

Index